Your

BEST WAY

to

Health

A Biblical-Medical Primer for Better Health

by

David L. Moore, M.D.

Published by: BEST WAY to Health, Inc.,
                  P.O. Box 463
                  Conyers, GA 30012
Cover design: Stacey Arndall
Layout: David L. Moore, M.D.
Editors: Shannan C. Moore, Patricia M. Smith,
                  M.A.
Printed in: United States of America
ISBN: 0-9678916-0-4

Scriptural Texts from the King James Version of the Bible.
Copyrighted material has been properly credited.

The material found in this book is for information purposes only and is not intended to be used in the diagnosis or treatment of any medical condition. All health concerns, should be evaluated by your primary care physician or other health professional. If you desire better health, follow the principles outlined in this primer. May God bless you as you take care of HIS TEMPLE, your body.

Dedicated to:

My father, the late Dr. Richard V. Moore whose example and love provided a role model which few sons have been privileged to have!

My mother, Mrs. B. J. Moore who initially suggested that I write this book! She has supported, encouraged and prayed for me throughout the years. Her love for me and all nine of her children, has been unfailing, just like Jesus.

My wife, Pam, who is the greatest blessing any husband could ever have, whom I love dearly.

Shannan and Emily, daughters who have been a constant joy. The best daughters a father could have.

My Lord and Savior Jesus Christ for His mercies and love. To Him be the praise and honor for the blessings received, through reading this book!

Special Thanks to:

My sister, Mrs. Patricia E. Smith, for the assistance, support, and encouragement given in the writing of this primer.

Mrs. Mamie E. Farmer, my mother-in-law, who has always provided encouragement and support for over 20 years, the best mother-in-law any son-in-law could have!

Connie Flint, Franz Lynch, Esmond Patterson and my WAOK family, whose encouragement and support have been such a blessing.

My Lifestyle Principles family for their support and prayers.

The Table of Contents

PREFACE

One of the most sought-after treasures in life, is good health. Time, energy, and money are spent to obtain this precious but elusive commodity. There are so many voices in the wind, touting, "this is the way." "Take this and it will alleviate all your problems!" "There's this new herb, it's great!" "You need this special vitamin formula!" So many products that promise so much but delivers so little, are the norms rather than the exception.

With multitudes of alternative therapies, legions of health care providers, myriads of philosophies, and almost endless treatment options; most of the public is confused as to where to turn, or who to believe.

Because medical science changes daily, it cannot be considered totally reliable. Consequently, there is a need for a source of dependable information upon which to base your beliefs. The Holy Scriptures are that source. God's Word, the source of all true knowledge, gives principles by which we are to live; a litmus test, if you will, to weigh all of life's issues. Therefore, you will find many Biblical quotations. Scientific research is also an essential component of this primer, with studies from reputable health journals and books referenced throughout.

Written from a unique Biblical-medical prospective, this book is design to be read by all who are interested in their health. You will appreciate its simple and straightforward approach, whether you have extensive or little medical knowledge. The principles you gain from this primer can form the basis for a lifetime of better health. The Biblical-medical approach, will also increase your faith in the Word of God while improving your health.

As a general practitioner who has practiced preventive lifestyle medicine for nearly twenty years, the author draws from the medical knowledge and practical experience he has gained to give you sound, simple, and practical information on health, which cannot be controverted. Some of the recommendations may be a little more rigorous than you are currently willing to follow. That's OK! Comply with those that are doable, and you will receive great benefits. But the closer these principles are followed, the better the results.

In an effort to make your reading more enjoyable and less monotonous, touches of humor, an integral part of the presentation style of the author, are used. Interspersed throughout the book, you will find little ☺ faces. So when you see them, you are suppose to smile! I trust this will be the case.

It is my hope that as you read, **Your "BEST WAY" to Health,** you will see practical ways in which you may honor God, through caring for His Temple, your body. May God's richest blessings be with you, so that you may discern and appreciate His way, which is, **Your "BEST WAY" to Health!**

PLEASE READ THE PREFACE BEFORE STARTING THIS BOOK!

CHAPTER 1

The Origin of Health

> *"And God saw every thing that he had made, and, behold, it was very good." Genesis 1:31*

Contrary to popular scientific research and belief, man did not evolve from lower forms of life. We are taught by many in the educational institutions of our land that evolution is a **fact**, and in the same breath, it is called the **theory** of evolution. One aspect of this theory that troubled me even as a child was, why aren't we still witnessing apes becoming humans, monkeys becoming apes, and aquatic animals becoming amphibians? When was the last time you witnessed a fish evolve into an alligator, or an ape becoming a man? An even more basic issue is, where did the earth come from in the first place? And if you accept the "Big Bang theory" where did the two large bodies originate that collided causing the "bang?" Even as a child I knew this theory was totally suspect and possibly erroneous.

7

totally suspect and possibly erroneous.

Another commonly accepted belief is that good health is just a stroke of luck, determined by what type of protoplasm we inherited from our parents. When people get sick, many say, "It was just in the cards I was dealt," as if they had no control over their own destinies. And while I know that heredity contributes to many of the illnesses we encounter, I also know that more than luck is involved in determining our health status.

Optimal health has its origin in a loving God, who with His own hands, formed us in His image. In the first chapter of Genesis we read, *"And God said, Let us make man in our image, after our likeness."* As Adam came from the Creator's hands, he was faultless. There was not one physical defect, illness did not exist, no blemishes marred his being. He was flawless in form, symmetry, statute, and intellect. No genetic mutations existed. Every cell, every chromosome, and every gene functioned flawlessly.

There was no stress for our first parents. Interpersonal relationships were ideal. No scolding words or venomous attacks were uttered by that blessed couple. God had ordained their union and had performed their marriage. He was first in their lives, and where God is first, there is peace and happiness. Adam and his wife lived harmoniously with every creature, great and small. There was no violence, only total harmony throughout all of creation.

The environment was pure. No pollution marred the air, land, or water. The atmospheric temperature and pressure were ideal. Neither pests, nor acid rain, nor harmful bacteria, nor viruses or fungi endangered the health or lives of plant or animal. The glorious sunlight penetrated and invigorated the air, warming the skin of our first parents. It's rays producing the vitamin D, which is essential in the development and maintenance of strong bones, teeth, and a healthy immune system.

Man's diet was given him by God and was only good. In fact, it too was ideal. The fruits, nuts, and grains were flawless in color, form, and taste. Every nutrient, macro and micro, was present in the appropriate amounts. There was no rancid or decaying vegetation to cause illness or disease. No animals or their potential offsprings were killed for man's food or for the food of other animals. The vegetation supplied man and animal with its life-giving properties.

The water was pristine, refreshing the most intense thirst and satisfying the needs of every cell in the bodies of man and animal.

Adam and Eve lived in a breathtaking home. A ceiling of matchless blue crowned their dwelling. The walls were of the most elegant foliage and included flowers more beautiful than any now in existence. The floor was carpeted with the softest, greenest, and most plush grass.

Though Adam and Eve had to work, they loved their job of dressing and keeping the garden. Our feeble minds cannot grasp its beauty or the pleasure they enjoyed in doing their daily "chores." They did not have weeds, thorns, pest, stones, rocks, or infertile soils in their garden home.

9

But most importantly, Adam and Eve enjoyed a perfect relationship with their Creator, talking with Him face to face and learning the secrets of life from the Source of all life. This was God's plan for our first parents. It is also His ultimate plan for each one of us. He want us to enjoy better health, even today, for He says in His word that, *"I wish above all things that thou mayest prosper and be in health." (3 John 2).*

But doesn't it seem strange, when you think about it, that the Omnipotent God, the Creator and Sustainer of the universe is **WISHING?** If you had all power, why would you have to wish for anything? You could just create whatever you desired. But the loving Creator of man and the universe has given you and I the freedom of choice. If you choose to obey Him, you can. This pleases Him and gives Him joy because He only wants what is best for you. If you choose not to obey, He will not force you too; even though He knows you will suffer the consequences of your actions. But because He loves you, He permits you to make mistakes and to learn from them. But know this: He is always eager, ready, and willing to forgive and forget. He loves you enough to allow you to make your own choices for time and for eternity. But oh, how much better for you, if you choose His way. Because it is the **"BEST WAY!"**

CHAPTER 2

Why Sickness, Disease and Death

"...Sir, didst not thou sow good seed in thy field? from whence then hath it tares? He said unto them, An enemy hath done this . . . " Matthew 13:27,28

The perfect home of our first parents was forfeited because of the choice Adam and Eve made when they were tempted by that, *"old serpent, called the Devil and Satan." (Rev. 12:19)* But where did sin and Satan come from? How did Lucifer, the covering cherub, the most exalted being ever created, become evil? For years I have contemplated these very difficult questions and have come up with very simple answers.

The law of God has always existed, because without laws you can have neither order nor government. And because there is in God's Ten Commandments, a **"thou shalt not,"** it automatically produces the possibility that, **"I shall."** Lucifer, and the fallen angels chose to exercise the "I shall," in spite of the plain "thou shalt not." This decision produced Satan. He then tempted Adam and Eve. The narrative of the first sin committed on planet Earth is as follows.

> *"Now the serpent was more subtle than any beast of the field which the Lord God had made. And he said unto the woman, Yea, hath God said, Ye shall not eat of every tree of the garden? And the woman said unto the serpent, We may eat of the fruit of the trees of the garden: But of the fruit of the tree which is in the midst of the garden, God hath said, Ye shall not eat of it, neither shall ye touch it, lest ye die. And the serpent said unto the woman, Ye shall not surely die: For God doth know that in the day ye eat thereof, then your eyes shall be opened, and ye shall be as gods, knowing good and evil. And when the woman saw that the tree was good for food, and that it was pleasant to the eyes, and a tree to be desired to make one wise, she took of the fruit thereof, and did eat, and gave also unto her husband with her; and he did eat. And the eyes of them both were opened, and they knew that they were naked; and they sewed fig leaves together, and made themselves aprons." (Gen.3:1-7)*

Our first parents chose of their own volition to believe a created being rather than the Creator. They knew what God had commanded, that He had created them, that He loved them, and that He had provided for them, yet they sought that which God knew was not best for them. They DISOBEYED and we see and live the inevitable consequences of that decision every day. Let's take a look at what they forfeited because of their choice.

1. They lost their beautiful home: *"Therefore the Lord God sent him forth from the garden of Eden, to till the ground from whence he was taken." (Gen.3.23)*
2. They forfeited their stress-free job: *"And unto Adam He said, Because thou hast hearkened unto the voice of thy wife, and hast eaten of the tree, of which I commanded thee, saying, Thou shalt not eat of it: cursed is the ground for thy sake; in sorrow shalt thou eat of it all the days of thy life; Thorns also and thistles will it brings forth to thee; and thou shalt eats the herb of the field; In the sweat of thy face shalt thou eat bread," (Gen.3: 17-19)*
3. Their marriage suffered as they sought to justify themselves. *"And the man said, The woman whom thou gamest to be with me, she gave me of the tree, and I did eat." (Gen.3: 12)*
4. But most importantly they lost their oneness with God: *"And they heard the voice of the Lord God walking in the garden in the cool of the day: and Adam and his wife hid themselves from the presence of the Lord God amongst the trees of the garden. And the Lord God called unto Adam, and said unto him, Where art thou? And he said, I heard thy voice in the garden, and I was afraid, because I was naked; and I hid myself." (Gen.3:8-10)*

Disobedience caused disorder. Disorder led to mutations in the genes of the cells of every living organism. These mutations were followed by diseases of every type. And disease resulted in death. Bacteria which at one time served a useful and constructive purpose became virulent, destructive and deadly!

Stress arose in the marriage and home of Adam and Eve, leading to disharmony and the detrimental physiologic changes, the "fight or flight response," which is the fruitful source of many of the diseases we face today.

The environment underwent changes so that protective clothing had to be worn. Droughts, famine, snow storms, hurricanes, tornados, and disasters occurred causing the lost of property, health, and life. The vegetation which once nourished man and animal changed, resulting in the growth of poisonous plants, weeds, thorns, and briars. Insects, once a positive component of creation became pests. They began destroying plants, and became a constant source of irritation to man and animal through their venomous and sometimes deadly bites and stings. Some of the animals became aggressive and ferocious attacking and killing other animals and even man, who at one time had total dominion over them.

Man began to WORRY about his food, his family, his health and even his relationship to God. OH, WHAT A DIFFERENCE ONE CHOICE MAKES!

But a loving God who says, *"I have loved thee with an everlasting love,"* *(Jer. 31:3)* did not leave man without hope. He placed in their bodies a defense, the immune system, which protected them from destructive internal and external forces. A system which, if kept in "tip-top" shape, will prevent the premature deaths of millions every year. Our job is to obey God's laws of love, both physical and moral. In fact, disease has been appropriately defined as "an effort of nature to free the system from conditions that result from a violation of the laws of health." *(E.G. White, Ministry of Healing. P.127, 1905)*

As you live in conformity to God's health laws, you will be less likely to become sick. But when sickness occurs, it is best to correct those lifestyle habits which caused the illness in the first place, rather than just being concerned about relief from the symptoms. Practically every day I am confronted with patients, whose only desire is that I, "make them feel better." "Doc, please keep me well, while I kill myself."☺ I have no problem with assisting my patients with symptom relief because that is one of my professional responsibilities. But many of the patients have little interest in addressing the cause of the problem and thus they become recurrently and perpetually ill. Let's suppose I offered you a job, and it was your responsibility to keep the floor in the restroom dry. A stopper is in the sink, the water is running and has started to overflow causing the floor to be wet. I hand you a mop and a bucket and say in a very pleasant tone, "Well, get to work." Talk about job security! ☺ But you would soon become tired of this, and would confront me with the "rocket science" solution of turning the water off, removing the stopper and then mopping the floor. This would be the best solution to this problem.

It is my hope that as you read this primer, you will be blessed of God to grasp His divine principles, turn off the water; apply them in your personal life, remove the stopper, so that better health may be realized in you life. As you do this, you will enjoy the more abundant life that Christ came to give, and eternal life when He comes again.

CHAPTER 3

The Source of Healing

> *"...for I am the LORD that healeth thee." (Ex. 15:26)*

In these simple words are outlined a truth that is often forgotten, ignored, or denied by many. Healing is attributed to the education and skill of man. And while man has a very important part to play in the process, all true healing comes from God. Modern medical advancements are accomplishing feats that were not even imaginable three decades ago. The ability to surgically separate siamese twins, to reattach severed limbs, and to transplant almost any organ of the body are all wonderful achievements; yet without the healing power of God, none of this could be accomplished. And now, with the ability to clone, man thinks "he's all that."☺ But with all our knowledge, we cannot perpetually cause the heart to beat, the lungs to breathe, or hair to grow! We cannot turn one gray hair black, permanently, even with all of our dyes.☺ Does the heart beat, or the lungs breathe by our will? These functions are all gifts from our Creator and are to be guarded as a sacred trust.

When you sustain a cut or injury, the healing power of God is immediately mobilized to stop the bleeding, prevent infection and begin the process of laying down new tissue and skin to repair the wound. This is a process that man with all of his knowledge and skill cannot duplicate. We may be able to remove a diseased gallbladder, but we cannot produce a new one. Only by the power of God, does the immune system fight off viral, fungal, and bacterial infections. Only by God's power can the body recuperate from a burn wound, from cancer, or even from a simple cold. What man attempts, is made possible by the power of a loving God!

Therefore, when you are confronted with any health issue you should go to the Great Physician, for His guidance, direction, and healing. He will direct you to the health practitioner that would best meet your needs should medical attention be necessary. He will also instruct you as to what questions to ask. When recommendations are given by the medical practitioner, He will let you know if that advice is best for you! Many have been instructed to follow a program which would be detrimental to them, and God has impressed them to question those recommendations; only to be informed that they had misunderstood the instructions. Sometimes a mistake was made and the wrong medication or treatment plan was given. God assures you that, *"I will instruct thee and teach thee in the way which thou shalt go: I will guide thee with mine eye."* *(Psalms.32.8)* When you depend on Christ for everything, He promises, *"I will never leave thee, nor forsake thee."* *(Heb. 13:5)*

If this is true, then why do so many people that believe in God get sick and die? This is a question that has troubled millions through the ages. God's Word has the answer. *"For the wages of sin is death." "All have sinned an come short of the glory of God." "Wherefore, as by one man sin entered into the world, and death by sin; and so death passed upon all men, for that all have sinned":* *(Romans 6:23, 3:23, 5:12)* The natural consequence of sin is sickness and death, as surely as the natural consequence of placing your hand on a hot stove is being burned. So no matter how "good" you are, you will experience pain, sickness, and will eventually die unless you live to see Jesus coming in the clouds. But you can reduce the probability of illness by giving heed to the simple instructions found in the Scriptures.

But I must remind you that for every authentic instruction that is found in God's word, Satan has legions of counterfeits. 2 + 2 = 4, one right answer. How many wrong answers are there? God's Word is truth, and Satan has a multitude of lies for each truth found in the Bible, one to suit your particular fancy. This is also true in the area of health. I see it daily. I will not attempt to describe every counterfeit that's out there; it would take volumes. Rather, I will do as I was taught when I worked in cash control at Walt Disney World. Due to the high volume of cash transactions that occurred at Walt Disney World in 1975, those of us who worked in that department were taught to identify counterfeit money. They never showed us even one, single, solitary, counterfeit bill! They taught us what things make a bill authentic, and knowing the true, made recognizing the counterfeit that much easier.

There are many perceived miracles of healing that are seen on television these days, but any healing without instructions on how to preserve health is only a short-lived experience, even if it is legitimate, which is another topic all together. (We will cover the area of counterfeits in health care later in this book.) Do you remember what Jesus told many after healing them? *"Go and sin no more."(John 8:11)* He realized that most illness is self-inflicted, caused by the way we live. If this was the way Jesus worked, then we should follow His example. In the next chapter we will look at some of the principles of health found in the Scriptures.

CHAPTER 4

"BEST WAY" the True Remedies

> *"But God hath chosen the foolish things of the world to confound the wise; and God hath chosen the weak things of the world to confound the things which are mighty..." 1 Corinthians 1:27*

The question is often asked, "how can I best maintain and/or improve my present health?" There are many methods that you can try, many voices in the wind. Some are just "plain-ole-bad." Some are good and others are better, but there is a **BEST WAY** which I'd like to share with you now.

BEST WAY is an acronym for the true remedies, which originate from our Creator, Jesus Christ.

20

Bedtime Regularity
Exercise
Sunshine and Simple Diet
Temperance

Water
Air
Yielding Trust in God

Each of these remedies was a part of man's original lifestyle in the Garden of Eden. I have studied medicine for more than 24 years and even with the significant medical discoveries, the outstanding technological advances, the plethora of new medications and surgical procedures, these remedies remain relevant. In fact, they will always be the foundation on which to build for a healthy lifestyle. Let's take a brief look at each of them.

BEDTIME REGULARITY

"It is vain for you to rise up early, to sit up late, to eat the bread of sorrows; for so he giveth his beloved sleep." (Psalms 127:2)

Scripture tells us that our God is a God of order. The certainty of the sun rising and setting, the tides of the ocean, and the orbit of the planets all demonstrate this fact. The Holy Spirit teaches us through Solomon that there is a time for everything under the sun. *(See Eccl. 3:1-8)* There is a time to sleep and a time to arise and work. As noted above He say in *Psalms 127:2, "It is vain for you to rise up early, to sit up late, to eat the bread of sorrows: for so he giveth his beloved sleep."*

It is best that you get at least seven hours of sleep each night. But with our highly stressed society, sleep disorders are increasing yearly. The number of over-the-counter preparations and prescription medications for sleep is steadily escalating. Medications are not best and should be avoided whenever possible. They may even be associated with an increased risk of death. A study in the journal, *Biological Psychiatry, March 1, 1998* reported a 29% increased mortality risk in those taking medications for sleep occasionally. There was an increased mortality of 65% in those taking medications more than 30 times per month. Most of these medications are also habit forming or addicting. Consequently sleeping pills are NOT the answer! I personally have never prescribed them for any of my patients.

Television is the vehicle which entices millions to stay up later than they should. This leads to an ever increasing number of medical problems related to inadequate sleep.

It has been said that two hours of sleep before midnight are as good as four hours after midnight. This is because of the normal circadian or bio-rhythms that our Creator placed in each one of us. The adage, "early to bed, early to rise makes a person healthy, wealthy, and wise" is true and should be practiced by all. Centenarians, those who live to be one hundred years old, usually work hard and sleep hard, getting at least 7-8 hours of sleep each day. The Adventist Health Study shows that sleeping 7-8 hours each night is associated with a longer life expectancy. So cut off the television and get to bed early, for your health.

The *Family Circle* magazine of January 6, 1998 revealed that sleep disorders affect almost 50% of all Americans, this is especially a problem in women. Inadequate sleep can make you irritable and can cause problems with concentration and decision making. Fatigue from inadequate sleep weakens the immune system causing a greater susceptibility to infections and other diseases.

In the *Harvard Mental Health Letter, August 1994*, it was noted that there are two types of sleep disorders: 1) An imbalance in the cycle of waking and sleeping; 2) A disorders in the sleep state. Difficulty sleeping occurs when the cues for adjusting our internal clock or bio-rhythms, have been distorted. And what are these cues? The main cue is light and darkness. God knew this, of course, and that's why we have day and night, light and darkness. But man has become a little god. We say, "let there be light" and we flip the switch and there is light. In our modern society with its artificial lights, this cue is definitely distorted. What can we do about this problem?

In the September issue of the same health letter, it was shown that properly timed light is an effective treatment for some sleep disorders, those caused by an imbalance in the sleep cycle. And for those with a disorder in the sleep state, intense artificial evening light during the day and early evening has been shown to reduce the risk of early morning awakening.

MELATONIN

Another recently discovered component in sleep physiology is the hormone melatonin. This hormone is produced by the pineal gland, a very small endocrine gland located at the base of the brain. It is produced in response to light stimulation. Melatonin will help to correct those sleep disorders that are due to disturbances associated with the light and darkness cycle. It has been demonstrated to be quite effective in the treatment of jet lag. It is interesting that our Creator placed in man's physiology the ability to produce proper amounts of melatonin if we will get proper exposure to light. This is why I recommend out-of-doors exercise during the morning. It leads to the production of more melatonin. *(Reiter RJ. The ageing pineal gland and its physiological consequences. Bioessays 1992 Mar; 14(3):169-175.)* There are also foods which increase melatonin production, oats, corn, rice, tomatoes, and bananas, to mention a few. Factors that decrease melatonin production include: stress, caffeine, alcoholic beverages, and tobacco. Some medications also decrease the production of melatonin, they include the non-steroidal inflammatory drugs (ibuprofen, naproxen, ECT.), anti-anxiety drugs, calcium channel blockers, beta blockers, vitamin B-12 supplements and antidepressants. *(Nedley, N M.D., Proof Positive, 1998, p.206)*

A genetic predisposition to sleep disorders has also been identified. "Abnormal sleep precedes the first episode of depression in people from families with a history of abnormal sleep profiles." *(Dr. Donna Giles, 12th. Annual Meeting of the Associate Professional Sleep Societies, June 12, 1998.)*

Often, I encourage patients to read the Bible if they can't sleep. One of two things will happen, either you will fall to sleep or you will get closer to God. A "no-lose" situation! ☺

So to get a good night's sleep, I suggest you follow the simple and practical steps listed in the "Ten Commandments for Sleep." They will help to insure you of a restful and rejuvenating night's sleep.

THE TEN COMMANDMENTS FOR GETTING A GOOD NIGHT'S SLEEP

1. Thou shalt have a regular schedule for going to and getting out of bed.
2. Thou shalt not take naps unless they are consistent, on a daily basis.
3. Thou shalt exercise regularly (daily if possible, preferably in the mornings.)
4. Thou shalt avoid caffeine in all forms (coffee, tea, chocolate, soft drinks.)
5. Thou shalt not use alcoholic beverages! They may help you fall to sleep but they distort the regular sleep cycle.
6. Thou shalt not take sleeping pills. Try a herbal tea like hops, scullcap or valerian.
7. Thou shalt find the best room temperature for you to sleep in. (Most people sleep better in a cool room.)
8. Thou shalt relax before going to bed. Take a warm bath, read a calming book, listen to soothing music and avoid stressful thoughts.
9. Thou shalt **NOT** eat heavily before going to bed.
10. Thou shalt trust God to give you the sleep you need.

EXERCISE

> *"And the Lord God took the man and put him into the garden of Eden to dress it and to keep it." (Genesis 2:15)*

WARNING: Please consult your physician before you begin an exercise program it you are over 40 years old or if you have a medical problem.

You were created to be an active being just like the Creator Himself. Your nervous, musculoskeletal, gastrointestinal, cardiovascular, and respiratory systems were made to accommodate physical activity. Originally, man was placed in the garden of Eden and given the job of cultivating the vegetation. This required the use of practically every part of his body and entailed the expenditure of energy. We term this, exercise.

Regular exercise has many psychological and physiological benefits. During exercise, respiration and circulation are improved, mental alertness is heightened, the muscles are strengthened, and the utilization of blood glucose by muscles is enhanced. These changes have a very beneficial effect in the treatment of certain disease processes.

Hypertension, or high blood pressure, is improved by exercise. Medical research has proven that with regular exercise the blood pressure can be lowered by 10 points in the systolic and diastolic pressures, after nine months of regular exercise. These results were seen in overweight 45-year-old men who were sedentary. *(American Journal of Hypertension; 1998:11:1405-1412)*

It is reported that 30% of Americans get no physical activity outside of their regular work. *(Morbidity & Mortality Weekly Report 1998;47:1097-1100)* The incidence of chronic diseases like heart disease, diabetes, and colon cancer is greater in those who are sedentary when compared to those who are physically active.

Diabetes mellitus, an elevation in the blood glucose or blood sugar, can be improved and even cured with regular physical exercise in tandem with a proper diet. Researchers at the University of Pittsburgh Medical Center, have shown that a 7-day exercise program decreased insulin resistance, leading to better blood glucose control. *(Hypertension, December 9, 1997)* Decreased insulin resistance is associated with a reduced risk of heart disease and strokes. This same effect was also seen in older Americans as reported in, *The Journal of the American Geriatrics Society, 1998;46:875-879.* The researchers observed a 25% improvement in the metabolism of glucose in those who exercised when compared to those that did not. So for diabetes, exercise is definitely helpful.

Exercise has a beneficial effect on the heart, and must be a component of any cardiac rehabilitation program. Exercise increases the HDL, "helpful" cholesterol, preventing blockages in the arteries. The mechanism through which this is accomplished is thought to be due to a decrease in the production of testosterone, as reported by Anthony C. Hackney of the University of North Carolina, Chapel Hill.

Another benefit of exercise is that it helps prevent osteoporosis or bone loss. This is important in older Americans because of the high risk of hip fractures associated with osteoporosis. To prevent this, older Americans are advised to remain physically active. Consuming adequate vegetables, calcium, and discontinuing tobacco use also help to prevent this problem. *(American Journal of Epidemiology 1998;147:871-879)* Patients with certain forms of arthritis are also benefitted by appropriate exercise.

Depression and anxiety are definitely improved with exercise. *(The Physician and Sports Medicine; Vol. 26; No. 10; October 98).*

Regular exercise helps to prevent, "middle-age spread" as reported in the *American Journal of Clinical Nutrition 1998;68:1136-1142.* Obese sedentary men over the age of 46 years old, were placed on an exercise program for six months. No dietary changes were made. The results, these men loss and average of 18 pounds. Even mild to moderate exercise, 10 minutes each day, was beneficial.

Animal studies document the benefits of exercise on the learning ability of laboratory mice. A twofold increase in the number of new brain cells appears in the areas of the brain responsible for learning in mice that were exercised versus those that were not. *(Nature Neuroscience; 1999: February)*

What are the best exercises? I believe that walking and useful labor (gardening, raking, vacuuming, etc.) are best. Seek to get at least twenty or more minutes of exercise, four of more times each week. While getting it all in one session is good, five or ten minute sessions totaling 20 or more minutes, is also advantageous. Even low intensity exercise is healthful. It is easy to see why our Creator placed man in a garden. It was a blessing to them and it will be a blessing to you.

SUNSHINE

"But unto you that fear my name shall the Sun of righteousness arise with healing in his wings:" (Malachi 4:2)

One of the most maligned and misunderstood of all the natural remedies is sunshine. I know people who are afraid to spend any time in the sun without a sunscreen. While we are aware that excessive amounts of sun exposure can be detrimental, everyone can benefit from appropriate amounts of sunshine. And isn't it just like the Devil to cause us to fear that which is best? And in some minds, if the *sun* is dangerous, then maybe the *Son* is dangerous too!

Appropriate sun exposure is beneficial in that it causes your body to convert cholesterol into a precursor of vitamin D. This vitamin is helpful in producing and maintaining strong bones and teeth. Studies in the journal, *Preventive Medicine 1993 Jan.;22 (1):132-140*, concluded, after reviewing articles from the past 50 years, that regular sun exposure is associated with significant decreases in death rates from certain cancers and a decrease in the overall cancer death rate. In addition these studies demonstrate the following:

1) Sunlight is the most effective source of vitamin D.
2) Regular sun exposure inhibited the growth of breast and colon cancer cells, and substantially reduced the rate of these cancers. In the magazine, *Your Health, April 1992;31(7):9-11*, it was reported that more than 15 minutes of sunshine each day can increase your risk of certain skin cancers which only occasionally caused death. But because vitamin D, produced by the sun is an

important mineral in the function of your immune system, women in the sunniest parts of the United States have the lowest rates of breast cancer, 1.5 times lower than women in northern cities like New York, Detroit, Boston, and Columbus, Ohio. Moreover, among workers at Western Electric Company in Chicago, those who got more than 150 IU of vitamin D per day only developed one half the colon cancer of those that got less. The recommended daily allowance (RDA) of vitamin D is 200 IU. **Ten to twenty minutes of direct, moderate sunlight on your arms or back per day produces 400 IU of vitamin D.**

3) Metabolites of vitamin D causes differentiation of leukemia and lymphoma cells. These changes prolonged the patient's life.

4) Long-term, regular, moderate sun exposure inhibits melanoma. Severe, recurrent sunburns initiated melanoma, the deadliest form of skin cancer.

5) Moderate, **infrequent** sun exposure is associated with an increase mortality rate for those cancers which have a 0.3% death rate. This accounts for approximately 2,000 deaths each year. But moderate **consistent** sun exposure helps to prevent other cancers with a death rate of 20-65%, which accounts for 138,000 fatalities in the United States annually.

6) Some scientists believe that the 17% increase in breast cancer is due to the anti-sun advisories given over the preceding 10 years.

7) Trends noted in the medical literature suggest that 30,000 U.S. cancer deaths could be prevented each year if the public adopted moderate, regular sun exposure.

8) Sunlight helps to prevent and counteract mental depression.

9) Sunlight helps us to sleep better due to the production of melatonin when the eyes are exposed to the sunlight particularly in the morning.

10) In the December 1996 *International Journal of Eating Disorders*, overweight women who were exposed to bright lights responded by showing improvement in their mood and in their weight. This finding shows that sunlight affects the melatonin-serotonin system, which is important in sleep and emotional physiology. It is also important in carbohydrate regulation.

11) Vitamin D also has a role in the prevention of prostate cancer. *(Women's Health Advocate Newsletter 1998 Feb.;4(12):1,8)*

12) Sunlight lowers blood pressure. *(Natures Banquet by Living Springs Retreat, p.100.)*

13) Sunlight reduces blood cholesterol by converting it to a precursor of Vit. D. (Ibid.)

14) Sunlight lowers blood sugar. (Ibid.)

15) Sunlight increases the body's resistance to infections. (Ibid.)

16) Sunlight raises the oxygen-carrying capacity of the red blood cells. (Ibid.)

17) Sunlight helps to balance the body's hormones. (Ibid.)

18) Sun exposure also kills viruses, bacteria, and fungi. This helps to prevent infections caused by these organisms.

So let's get some sun! It could save your life. And get THE SON; HE will not only save your life but will give you eternal life!

SIMPLE DIET

"And God said, Behold, I have given you every herb bearing seed, which is upon the face of all the earth, and every tree, in the which is the fruit of a tree yielding seed; to you it shall be for meat." (Genesis 1:29)

In our complex society, it's hard to believe that the simple things in life are, in fact, the best. The Gospel, for instance, is a simple contract. We recognize our sinfulness and our total inability to save ourselves from sin's penalty. Through the workings of the Holy Spirit, we believe that Jesus Christ paid the penalty for our sins through His death on the cross. We accept this gift and He gives us eternal life! This is the Gospel. This life saving, life giving, dynamic process is very simple, but very true.

When it comes to diet, God has provided what He knows is best for the bodies He created. If you owned a Lexus and it needed servicing, you would not take it to a Yugo mechanic, even if you could find one.☺ (Yugos were neither reliable nor well-constructed automobiles and are no longer imported to the United States.) You would instead, take your Lexus to someone who was qualified to service it. And who is more qualified than those who made it. The same is true in reference to your body. God created you and He knows what foods are best for you. In Genesis chapter one, verse twenty-nine, we read: *"And God said, Behold, I have given you every herb bearing seed, which is upon the face of all the earth, and every tree, in the which is the fruit of a tree yielding seed; to you it shall be for meat."* This is the diet which God chose, and it is best. Today, we term this a vegetarian or vegan diet.

Medical science for centuries has repeatedly pronounced God's original diet for man as inadequate in protein, certain minerals, and vitamins. But the more we learn about diet and nutrition, the more we understand that God knew what He was doing when he gave man his diet. The original diet was composed of fruits, grains, and nuts. Later vegetables were added after man sinned. This diet would be described as a high complex carbohydrate, adequate protein, and low fat diet. Man was not allowed to eat flesh meats until after the flood destroyed all vegetation. The life expectancy dropped by over 600 years when you compare the ten generations before and the ten generations after the flood. The Bibles records, *"And all the days that Adam lived were nine hundred and thirty years: and he died." (Genesis 5:5) "And Reu lived two and thirty years, and begat Serug: And Reu lived after he begat Serug two hundred and seven years, and begat sons and daughters." (Genesis 11:20,21)* We see that a drastic reduction in the life expectancy took place. I believe that diet had a great deal to do with this change. Recent studies demonstrate that flesh foods are associated with an increase incidence of prostate cancer *(Journal of the National Cancer Institute 1999;91:414-428)*, heart disease *(British Medical Journal, April 3, 1998)* and food poisoning from salmonella, e. coli, and other disease causing bacteria. Flesh meats are more of a threat to health today than ever before because of the diseases found in animals. The fact that God did not include them in the original diet of man lets us know that they are not essential neither are they the best foods for us.

Let's compare the food pyramid proposed by the United States Department of Agriculture in 1992 (a vegetarian version) with man's original diet.

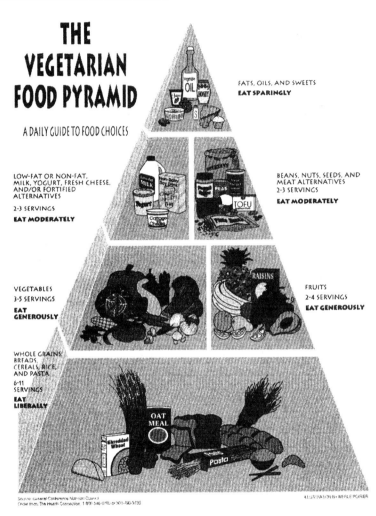

The food pyramid recommends that you get 6-11 servings of whole grains in the form of breads, cereals, rice and pasta each day, all complex carbohydrates. These whole grains contain vitamin E, which prevent clotting; complex carbohydrates, which act as a source of energy; and fiber, which is so important in the function of the digestive system and also in cholesterol metabolism.

It also recommends that you consume 5-10 servings of fruits and vegetables each day. These foods are primary sources of important vitamins including, B, A, C, folate, and K. In addition they are the principal sources of a newly discovered group of nutrients called phytochemicals. These chemicals are known to help prevent and treat infections, cancers, hypertension, and heart disease, just to name a few. Fruits and vegetables are also excellent sources of potassium, which is very important in cellular metabolism. A high potassium intake is also associated with lower blood pressures. The phytochemical lycopene found in tomatoes helps to prevents cell damage caused by free-radicals. Free radicals are byproducts of metabolism which damages normal cells, causing them to become cancerous. *(American Journal of Clinical Nutrition 1999; 69:712-718)*

The following table lists some of the known phytochemicals, their source and action.

PHYTOCHEMICALS	POSSIBLE ACTION	FOOD SOURCE
Allicin, allylic sulfides	Detoxifies bacteria (possibly H. pylori an ulcer causing agent), reduces cholesterol levels	Onions, garlic, scallions, leeks, chives
Capsaicin	Reduces low-density (LDL) cholesterol, prevents carcinogen activation, detoxifies carcinogens (cancer causing agents)	Strawberries, raspberries, other berries
Chlorogenic acid	Blocks nitrosamines formation (a potent carcinogen)	Tomatoes, green peppers, pineapples
Flavonoids (4,000 different compound including flavonols, isoflavones, and flavones)	Antioxidants, reduce cell overgrowth, helps remove carcinogens from cells, prevents bone thinning, soy isoflavones lower total and LDL cholesterol	Widely distributed in fruits and vegetables
Indoles	Helps enzymes to form estrogen; thought to be protective against breast, colon, esophageal, prostate, and lung cancers.	Cabbage, broccoli, brussels sprouts, cauliflower, collards, kale, mustard greens, turnips, rutabaga
Limonoids	Increase production of protective proteins (enzymes)	Citrus fruits, particularly the rinds
Monoterpenes	Antioxidants	Broccoli, cabbage, citrus fruits, yams, cucumbers, eggplant, parsley, peppers, squash, tomatoes
P-Coumaric acid	Blocks production of cancer-causing nitrosamines during digestion	Tomatoes, green peppers, pineapple, strawberries
Protease inhibitors	Lengthen the time it takes for cancer cells to develop	Soybeans, cereals, beans
Triterenoids	Suppress the carcinogenic activity of estrogen	Soybeans, licorice root extract, citrus fruits, carrots

Adapted from Hospital Medicine. August 1998. Phytochemicals: the newest frontier in disease prevention; 56, A. Wolf, MS, RD and A. Wolf, MD.

The protein group on the food pyramid is composed of dairy products, flesh meats, eggs, nuts, and beans. Proteins should comprise only a moderate part of your diet with the daily intake restricted to 4-6 servings. In the early 1900's conventional wisdom dictated that we needed about 100 grams of protein each day. This is very difficult to obtain without consuming dairy products, eggs, and flesh meats. In 2000, we are certain that 40-50 grams of protein are best for optimal health. This amount is easily obtained in the diet of our first parents. We also know that a high protein diet is linked to kidney stones, certain cancers, atherosclerosis, and some immune system dysfunctions.

At the very top of the pyramid is the fat group. From it we should eat very sparingly. High dietary fat is associated with a greater incidence of breast, colon and prostate cancers. Diabetes mellitus, obesity, degenerative arthritis, gallbladder disease, coronary artery disease, immune system compromise, and hormonal abnormalities are also associated with a high fat intake. The original diet was definitely a low fat diet. Nuts were the primary source of fats along with avocados. Recently, it has been documented that nuts actually prevent atherosclerosis, which causes heart attacks and some forms of strokes.*(Annals of Internal Medicine 2000;132:538-546)*

BREAKFAST, A MUST!

Breakfast, the most important meal of the day, is the meal you eat upon arising from sleep and is the meal that is most often skipped. The reason for this is simple, we are not usually hungry in the morning, therefore we skip breakfast. Why? Usually because we have eaten too much in the evening. If the heavy suppers were omitted along with snacks, then a substantial breakfast would be eaten every morning! The importance of breakfast has been well documented in the medical literature. But more importantly, the Word of God indicates that God wants His children to eat a good breakfast every day. *"And Moses said, This shall be, when the LORD shall give you in the evening flesh to eat, and in the morning bread to the full; for that the LORD heareth your murmurings which ye murmur against him: and what are we? your murmurings are not against us, but against the LORD."* *(Exodus 16:8)* " *And the ravens brought him bread and flesh in the morning, and bread and flesh in the evening; and he drank of the brook."(1 Kings 17:6)*

A few of the known benefits of a good breakfast are:
1. Men who eat a good breakfast regularly have a 40% lower risk of dying than those who skip breakfast. Women who eat a good breakfast have a 30% lower risk.
2. Regular nutritious breakfasts improve a person's perception of his or her well-being. You feel better when you are in the habit of eating a good breakfast daily.
3. Those who eat a high complex carbohydrate breakfast, typically have more energy, less fatigue, and sleepiness than those who skipped breakfast. A high protein breakfast on the other hand, though it consists of the same number of calories, caused more fatigue and sleepiness.

4. Data from the New York Safety Council reveals that people who eat a warm breakfast are less likely to have a highway accident on the way to work compared to those who skip it. This is because missing breakfast causes an increase in reaction time, the amount of time it takes to react. In North Carolina, textile workers who skip breakfast accounted for 75% of the accidents that occur in that industry.

5. Skipping breakfast causes hunger that affects behavior. The behavior observed included a decrease in attentiveness, and an increase in hyperactivity, and irritability.

6. School performance is better in students who eat breakfast than those who did not.

7. Blood cholesterol levels are lowest among adults eating a nutritious breakfast daily that includes a high-fiber cereal. Those who skipped breakfast had the highest cholesterol levels.

8. Those eating nutritious breakfasts are more likely to eat balanced and nutritious meals the rest of the day.

9. The *Iowa Breakfast Study* reported that the omission of breakfast is of no advantage in a weight reduction program. **Those who omitted breakfast not only increased their hunger but also suffer a significant loss of efficiency in the late morning hours.**

10. A study conducted by the University of Minnesota established that part of the success in losing weight may depend upon when calories are eaten. Calories consumed early in the day are more likely to be used to support energy requirements. But those consumed late in the day or during the night, when the body temperature is falling, are stored as body fat, in order to keep the body temperature normal.

11. A study of 175 overweight women who were hospitalized continued to lose weight more than six months after leaving the hospital, if their calories **were not concentrated in the afternoon and evening.**

WHAT MAKES UP A GOOD BREAKFAST?

As mentioned earlier, a high complex carbohydrate breakfast is best. Adequate protein is also very important. A good breakfast should include a whole grain cereal with soy milk, three or four servings of fresh, canned, or dried fruit, and a couple of pieces of 100% whole grain bread with a little nut butter or a few nuts. This would provide all of the nutrients needed for the morning and early afternoon.

The best commercial dry cereals include:
1. Shredded Wheat
2. Total
3. Uncle Sam Cereal
4. Cheerios
5. Other whole grain cereals

Good hot cereals include:
1. Oatmeal (Quick or Old Fashion)
2. Barley Flakes
3. Millet
4. Grape Nuts or similar store brand cereals with soy milk. Cook for one minute in the microwave.
5. Fruit crisp. *

Other breakfast foods include:
1. Cashew-Oat waffles *
2. Potato cakes *
3. Scrambled tofu *
4. Granola *

41

Many prefer to eat their "dinner" foods for breakfast. This is fine, but omit all fatty foods. Eat more beans, whole grains, and vegetables; and eliminate meat totally, for optimal health.

★You will find the recipes for breakfast and other healthful dishes in the appendix.

I would now like to give you some guidelines that will enhance your physical, mental and even your spiritual health. While there is not a "one diet that fits all," these guidelines are quite comprehensive in scope, and will be of benefit in regaining and maintaining your health. The reason, it is based upon the Word of God.

WARNING: If you have diabetes or some other chronic medical condition, please consult your physician before you begin this dietary program.

THE PRUDENT DIET

These principles are given as a foundation upon which you may build a healthful diet.

WHEN TO EAT

Eating at regularly scheduled times is very important. Allow 5-6 hours between each meal! YOU SHOULD HAVE ABSOLUTELY NOTHING BETWEEN MEALS BUT WATER. The smallest meal should be the one before going to sleep. Eat nothing before going to sleep unless you want to toss and turn.☺ Heavy suppers and between meal snacks are the fruitful source of inappropriate growth, out but not up.☺ **OMIT THE THIRD MEAL IF YOU ARE TRYING TO LOSE WEIGHT!**

WHAT TO EAT

GRAINS: Use whole grain products. 100% whole grain bread is best. Brown rice is preferable to white rice. Other whole grains such as oats, rye, corn, barley, and millet are also important.

FRUITS: Choose fresh fruit in season instead of canned fruit when possible. When using canned fruits, use only those canned in juice and/or water. Do not use fruit in light or heavy syrup. This only adds calories to your diet, which most people do not need.☺ Dried fruit is also excellent. Five (5) servings of fruit every day contribute to optimal health.

NUTS: Eat nuts in moderation. Do not eat nuts alone because you will find it difficult to stop. Take it from me. I know!☺ Always make nuts a part of your meal. Almonds are excellent. Canned nuts with salt and oil should be

43

avoided.

OLIVES: Properly cured black or green olives are an excellent food. They are soothing to an inflamed or irritated stomach. Rinse canned olives several times, then soak them in water overnight in the refrigerator to avoid excess salt.

VEGETABLES: Eat a wide variety! Remember green leafy along with deep yellow vegetables. Raw salads are also excellent. Dark green leafy vegetables are excellent sources of calcium, iron, B-vitamins, and vitamin A. A high intake of vegetables is associated with a decreased risk of stomach cancer. *(American Journal of Epidemiology 1999;149:925-932)*

LEGUMES: These are beans, peas, and lentils. They contain proteins, fiber, complex carbohydrates, vitamins, minerals, a host of phytochemicals and a small amount of fats.

DAIRY: **It is best to dispense with the use of dairy products altogether.** They are generally high in fat. The lactose in dairy products may cause profound digestive difficulty. Soy products are far superior.

EGGS: Eggs are optional. A good replacement for scrambled eggs is scrambled tofu. (See the recipe in Appendix.) If you choose to use eggs, eat no more than 1-2 per week, due to the large amount of cholesterol found in the yoke.

SALT: Use only small amounts of salt when cooking. When shopping, buy foods with no added salt. Or try to limit the sodium content of the foods you buy to **no more than 175 mg. per serving**. A high sodium intake is associated with an elevated blood pressure in some individuals. Salty snacks are associated with an increased incidence of stomach cancer. *(American Journal of Epidemiology 1999;149:925-932)*

HOW TO PREPARE FOODS

Prepare foods as simply as possible, but make them attractive and appetizing. Boil, bake or broil! **DO NOT FRY**! Frying adds flavor to foods but it also adds calories which are not needed. In fact, ladies, the only thing you should use a frying pan for is to keep those males in your house in line. ☺ You should avoid shortening and other hard fats such as butter and stick margarine. Use vegetable oils sparingly because they are as high in calories as animal fats. Avoid spices and condiments that irritate the delicate stomach lining. If a substance is cold in the hand, and hot in the mouth, it should be avoided.☺ Nonirritating herbs like parsley, thyme, sweet basil, sage, onions, garlic, etc. are excellent as seasonings.

PROTEIN

There are many misconceptions about proteins and the body's need for them. While proteins are an essential element of your diet, the body actually uses the amino acids that make up the proteins in its functions. Amino acids are the alphabets, the proteins are the words. Your digestive system breaks down the ingested proteins into their constituent amino acids. These amino acids are then extracted from the bloodstream by the cells of your body as needed. It is important to keep the amino acid pool filled, which can easily be done on a vegetarian diet. The following food combinations make what is termed a COMPLETE PROTEIN (a protein having the right amounts and the right combination of the eight essential amino acids) when these foods are eaten within a thirteen-hour period.

1.   A whole grain and legumes (beans). Example: beans and brown rice.
2.   A whole grain and nuts. Example: 100% Whole wheat bread and peanut or any nut butter.

45

3.   Legumes and nuts. Example: Soy milk and almonds.

The soybean has been studied extensively and is called by some the "MIRACLE BEAN." I personally believe that the benefits of the soybean can be found in other beans also, but they have not been studied as extensively.

1.   Soybeans are an excellent source of calcium. Dr. Kironobu Katsuyama and colleagues at the Kawasaki Medical School in Japan states soybeans and their products may help to prevent osteoporosis.

2.   Soybeans are an excellent source of polyunsaturated fats which are associated with a reduction in heart disease and prostate cancer.

3.   Dr. Mark Jordinson and colleagues at the Imperial College School of Medicine in London, UK state that soybean lectins, a phytochemical, have an anti-tumor effect on cancer cells in mice.

4.   The use of soy milk instead of cows' milk is beneficial for almost everyone, especially those who are lactose intolerant.

5.   Soybeans are the only single plant source of a complete protein.

The soy products we use in my home are the **"Better Than Milk"** products, produced by Fuller Life Natural Foods in Maryville, Tn. They may be found in your local health food stores or supermarkets.

FATS

Fats contain two and one half times more calories than proteins or carbohydrates. In the United States, we consume far too many fats. Fats make up forty percent of the calories in the average American diet. Most nutritional authorities believe that no more than 30% of your calories should be derived from fat.

There are two types of fats: saturated and unsaturated. Hard fats such as butter, margarine, and lard are saturated. Unsaturated fats are mainly liquid or semi-solid at room temperature. One researcher, believes that the rapid increase in the incidence of cancer is the result of using more hydrogenated fats, unsaturated fat artificially made into a saturated fat by mechanically adding hydrogen to the molecule. *(Gabe Mirkin, M..D., Audio Digest Family Practice, Vol.47, Issue 26).* This process forms a trans fat, which is known to be detrimental to your body.

A high dietary fat intake is associated with an increase incidence of cancer of the beast, prostate, colon, and pancreas. Heart disease is also associated with a high dietary fat intake. While some believe that only saturated fats are bad for you, too much unsaturated fat will contribute to obesity, which is associated with Type 2 diabetes mellitus, hypertension, degenerative arthritis, and a host of other medical problems.

I believe it is best to restrict the total fat intake to no more than 20% of your total calories. The easiest way to reach this ideal is to make sure that only a few items in your diet contain more than 20% of their total calories in the form of fats. Example: when reading a food label, if the total calories in the food are 120 calories per serving, then the fat calories should be no more than 24 calories. If you follow this practice of counting fat calories you will maintain a low-fat diet which is best for your health.

SUGAR

Sugar, or sucrose is a highly maligned foodstuff because it is totally devoid of any significant nutrients and contains only, "empty calories." To metabolize this "food," the body's own stores of nutrients are taxed and even depleted. While a small amount of sugar is not all that bad, Americans are eating it in excessive amounts. The per capita intake of sugar in the United States is over 147 lbs. annually. This amount makes it the fruitful cause of many illnesses. *(Putnam JJ, Allshouse, JE. Food Consumption, Prices, and Expenditures, 1996. Statistical; Bulletin No. 928, US Dept. of Agriculture, P.20)*

I'm sure you are saying, "I don't eat that much sugar!" But you may be getting it from unsuspected sources. Manufacturers have become very creative in the way they camouflage sugar in foods. If you see, dextrose, cane sugar, corn sweetener, corn syrup, high fructose corn syrup, sucrose, glucose, sugars, or inverted sugar, all are just fancy names for sugar.

Eight cancers that are linked to our "normal" sugar consumption in the U.S. are, colon, rectal, breast, ovarian, uterine, prostate, kidney, and cancers of the nervous system. *(Armstrong B, Doll R. "Environmental factors and cancer incidence and mortality in different countries, with special reference to dietary practices." **International Journal of Cancer** 1975 April 15:15(4):617-631)*

The table below list the sugar content of common foods:

HIDDEN SUGARS IN FOODS

Food	Tsp. sugar
Malted milk (12 oz.)	42
Soft drinks (12 oz.)	10-12
Canned Fruit (light syrup)	8
Chocolate cake (4 oz.)	8
Chocolate candy (1 oz.)	7
Fruit pie (1 slice)	7
Ice Cream (1 scoop)	5
Donut, glazed	4
Jam, jelly (1 Tbsp)	3

(The Food Processor for Windows: Nutrition Analysis & Fitness Software. ESHA Research, Salem, Oregon.)

Sugar compromises the immune system like few other dietary substances. Consider the effects of sugar on the white blood cell's ability to destroy disease causing bacteria of your body.

SUGAR & WHITE BLOOD CELL FUNCTION

Teaspoons of sugar	*No. bacteria destroyed*
0	14.0
6	10.0
12	5.5
18	2.0
24	1.0

(Kijak E, Foust G, Steinman RR. *Relationship of blood sugar level and leukocytic phagocytosis*. Southern California Dental Association 1964:32(9):349-357)

It is my belief that this is the reason why so many colds, flu, and other infections occur around the Thanksgiving, Christmas and New Years holidays. During these times, sugar consumption is much higher because of the pies, cakes, candies and other sugar laden foods eaten during the holidays.

HOW TO EAT
Chew your food thoroughly and well. Do not wash food down with liquids. Eat enough to satisfy your hunger, and not your appetite or "desire." Overeating is a great enemy to proper physical and mental health. You need to use your digestive and not your respiratory system when you eat. Chew your foods well, don't inhale them!☺

WHEN NOT TO EAT
Do not eat right before or after strenuous physical or mental effort. Mild physical exercise, like a short walk, after a meal aids digestion and enhances the utilization of the calories that were just consumed. Do not eat a full meal when you are too rushed, tense, anxious, or worried. Eat less or skip that meal.

WATER
Water is the best beverage for quenching your thirst and is also the best liquid for cleansing body tissues. **DRINK 6-8 GLASSES EACH DAY.** Drink it a little time before or after meals. Do **NOT** drink water with your meals because this hinders digestion. With the epidemic gastric reflux disease there is no need of making matters worst.☺ Only drink water between meals.

SUMMARY

Have a regular time to eat your meals each day. Eat a good breakfast every day and reduce or eliminate suppers, unless you are trying to gain weight or keep from losing it. Let nothing come even close to your lips between meals except for air, water and your loved-one's lips.☺ Avoid eating fatty foods because of the excessive calories they contain. Eat a large quantity of fruits and vegetables every day, 5-10 servings. Make sure you eat beans as often as possible, and use whole grains instead of refined products. Remember *ECCLESIASTES 10:17 - "... Eat for strength and not for drunkenness."* May God bless you as you eat to glorify Him, and not to satisfy an undisciplined appetite!

TEMPERANCE

"And every man that striveth for the mastery is temperate in all things." I Corinthians 9:25

This is a term that has been misunderstood for centuries. The *World Book Dictionary 1989 Edition* defines temperance as, "the state or quality of being moderate in action, speech or habits; self-control. The state or quality of being moderate in the use of alcoholic drinks. The principle and practice of not using alcoholic drinks at all." While these are good definitions, true temperance means much more.

"True temperance teaches us to dispense entirely with everything hurtful and to use judiciously that which is healthful." (E. G. White, Patriarch and Prophets 1890, p.562) Temperance is very important in securing a healthful life here, and is vital as we seek to make heaven our home.

The Bible says, *"And every man that striveth for the mastery is temperate in all things." (1 Corinthians 9:25) "But the fruit of the Spirit is love, joy, peace, longsuffering, gentleness, goodness, faith, meekness, temperance: against such there is no law." (Galatians 5:22, 23)* Through intemperance Satan gained the victory over our first parents in the Garden of Eden. Victory over intemperance was the first gained by Christ when tempted in the wilderness. *(See Matthew 4: 1-4)*

Let's take a closer look at the above definition. It has two components. The first is total abstinence from everything known to be harmful, such as caffeine, tobacco in any form, alcoholic beverages, illegal drugs, and the misuse of prescription drugs. The second component requires you to use in moderation those things that are healthful. Whole wheat bread is healthful, but you would not eat two loaves at a meal.☺ Exercise is important but we should not overdo it. We have a tendency to either do too much or nothing at all. There must be balance. Overworking, oversleeping, overeating, overdoing anything is detrimental. A case in point, the *American Journal of Cardiology 1998;81:1243-1245* revealed that mowing the lawn with a manual or push mower taxed heart patients causing a myocardial infarct, or heart attack.

If you apply this simple principle of temperance to your life, God's Word assures that you will be blessed with improved health.

CAFFEINE

This drug, though many may not think of it as a such, is consumed by millions the world over, and is considered an innocuous substance. But this is just not the case. Caffeine is found in practically all coffee, chocolate, dark-colored and even some light-colored soft drinks. All teas contain caffeine, with the exception of herbal teas. Please see the following chart for the caffeine content of some common "foods."

CAFFEINE CONTENT OF CERTAIN FOODS

BEVERAGES

	Serving Size	Caffeine (mg)
Coffee, drip	5 oz.	110-150
Coffee, perk	5 oz.	60-125
Coffee, instant	5 oz.	40-105
Coffee, decaffeinated	5 oz.	2-5
Tea, 5-minute steep	5 oz.	40-100
Tea, 3-minute steep	5 oz.	20-50
Hot cocoa	5 oz.	5-10
Cola	12 oz.	45

FOODS

Milk chocolate	1 oz.	1-15
Bittersweet chocolate	1 oz.	5-35
Chocolate cake	1 slice	20-30

OVER-THE COUNTER DRUGS

Anacin, Empirin, Midol	2	64
Excedrin	2	130
NoDoz	2	200
Aqua-Ban (diuretic)	2	200
Dexatrim (Wt. Control aid)	2	200

Adapted from The Wellness Encyclopedia, University of California, Berkeley, 1991:137, Houghton Muffin Co.

In one medical practice it was noted that a 7-year-old male had tics, twitches, of his neck and face. He was consuming 2 to 4 servings of caffeine containing products each day. When caffeine was eliminated for six months, the tics stopped. In another case, a 11-year-old male was experiencing tics for over two years. He was consuming 2-4 servings of caffeine containing products each day. When the caffeine was eliminated, the tics resolved in two weeks. *(Pediatric electronic pages 1998;101 (6):e4)*

Caffeine consumption before and during pregnancy is associated with an increased risk of fetal loss. *(JAMA, December 22/29, 1993-Vol. 270, No.24:2940)*. It is common knowledge that caffeine causes irritability, and when abruptly discontinued, leads to withdrawal symptoms, the most common being headaches. This is seen even in children.

Caffeine also can affect blood pressure. One cup of a caffeinated drink may raise the systolic and diastolic blood pressure five to six points. When consumed before exercise, caffeine raises the heart rate and blood pressure even more which may cause an increased risk in those with heart disease. *(Nedley, N. One Nation Under Pressure. Proof Positive, Neil Nedley, MD, p.142, Ardmore, OK)*. This is why Margo Wootan, a senior scientist for the watchdog group, Center for Science in the Public Interest wants manufacturers to list the caffeine contents of foods and drinks.

Coffee contains known carcinogens (cancer causing substances). Including: methylglyoxal, catechol, chlorogenis acid and neochlorogenic acid. Coffee may cause an increased risk of bladder cancer and a twofold increase in the death rate from the same cancer. *(Nedley, N. One Nation Under Pressure. Proof Positive, Neil Nedley, MD, p.30, Ardmore, OK)*.

Colon cancer death may be also related to coffee consumption. Those who drank more than two cups per day had a 70% increased risk of death from colon cancer compared to those who used coffee less than once per day. *(Snowdon, DA, Phillips, RL, Coffee consumption and the risk of fatal cancers, Am J Public Health 1984 Aug;74(8):820-823)*

Caffeine is a known stimulant and will definitely interfere with sleep. Those with a sleep disorder should avoid caffeine in all forms. It is not a bad idea to eliminate caffeine totally!

ALCOHOL & DRUGS

"Wine is a mocker and strong drink is raging; and whosoever is deceived thereby is not wise." (Pro. 20:1) "Who has woe? who hath sorrow? who hath contentions? who hath babbling? who hath wounds without cause? who hath redness of eyes? They that tarry long at the wine; they that go to seek mixed wine. Look not thou upon the wine when it is red, when it giveth colour in the cup, when it moveth itself aright. At the last it biteth like a serpent, and stingeth like an adder. Thine eyes shall behold strange women, and thine heart shall utter perverse things." (Proverbs. 23:29-33)

Here we find divine instructions to abstain from the use of wine and strong drink. All illegal drugs would fall into this injunction. The list of medical and social ills brought on by the use of illegal drugs and alcoholic beverages are numerous. While working in an urgent care center in Charlotte, NC I had the regrettable task of seeing many married men who either thought they had or did in fact have a sexually transmitted disease. Many were happily married and had been out of town on a business trip. I always asked them if they had been drinking. Ninety percent confessed that they had, which had lead to them being unfaithful. Most sincerely regretted their actions. This shows the validity of the above scriptures. When using alcoholic beverages or other drugs, a person loses practically all inhibitions which leads to regrettable actions and consequences.

Yearly, thousands are killed on our nations' highways because of the use of alcohol and drugs. The number of broken homes and "hearts" caused by the use of these substances are untold. Satan is seeking to destroy you and anyone he can through their use. No Christian should use alcoholic beverages, tobacco, or illegal drugs!

The scientific literature is filled with studies stating that wine is good for the heart and for circulation. But recent articles indicate that this benefit is coming from the grapes themselves and not from the fermented juice of the grapes. The use of purple grape juice is associated with changes that improves the circulation by causing vasodilation, and a reduction in the LDL (lousy) cholesterol. *(Stein, JH, Circulation 1999 100: 1050-1055)*. The sum effect being a reduction in the risk of heart disease.

The flavonoids in grapes, fruits, and vegetables help to prevent platelets from sticking together preventing the inappropriate clotting of the blood. These flavonoids are more powerful antioxidants than vitamin E. So it is clear that the supposed benefits of wine are just that, supposed and not actual. It's the grapes!

Moderate alcohol use may even raise the cancer risk in the upper digestive tract as reported in the *Medical Tribune,*

Family Practice Edition, Nov. 5,1998. Alcohol also has a direct effect on the diastolic and systolic blood pressures. It increases the blood glucose, total cholesterol, LDL (lousy) cholesterol, and triglycerides, all of which are harmful to the heart and circulatory system. *(Family Practice News, p.7, November 15, 1998)*

Satan cripples and at times destroys the unborn with this noxious brew. Fetal alcohol syndrome is all too prevalent today. And when mothers that breast fed their babies consumed even small to moderate amounts of alcohol, it altered the sleep patterns of their babies. It was noted by Drs. Julie A. Mennella and Carolyn J. Gerrish of the Monell Chemical Senses Center in Philadelphia, PA that infants who had alcohol tainted breast milk slept 25% less than those infants fed regular breast milk. Chronic sleep disturbances which occur while the infant's brain is trying to develop may cause learning disabilities. *(Pediatric electronic pages 1998;101-102)*

The World Health Organization says:

♦ "Alcohol consumption causes some of the world's most serious problems."
♦ "Drinking adversely effects a significant proportion of the population, not just a minority of alcoholics or heavy drinkers."
♦ Light drinking is unlikely to lower heart disease risk in people who are taking other lifestyle precautions like exercising regularly, not smoking, and eating less fat.
♦ The publicity given to the moderate use of alcohol for heart disease is "not the result of rigorous scientific research, but is to a large extent inspired by commercial purposes."
♦ "The less you drink, the better," is their recommendation.

ALCOHOL USE IN TEENAGERS

An entire generation is being assaulted by Satan through the use of alcohol and drugs. The table that follows was published in *The Family Practice News, November 1, 1998 p.45.* It displays an alarming incidence of drug experimentation and use among teens, even as young as 13 years old.

LIFETIME PREVALENCE OF DRUG ABUSE, 1997*

DRUG	8TH. Graders	10th. Graders	12th. Graders
Alcohol	53.8%	72.0%	81.7%
Cigarettes	47.3%	60.2%	65.4%
Marijuana	22.6%	42.3%	49.6%
Inhalants	21.0%	18.3%	16.1%
Stimulants	12.3%	17.0%	16.5%
LSD	4.7%	9.5%	13.6%
Cocaine	4.4%	7.1%	8.7%
Heroin	2.1%	2.1%	2.1%

*Data from the Monitoring the Future Study, which is based on a survey of 51,000 8th., 10th. , and 12th. grade students at 429 secondary schools across the United States.

It is easy to discern that Satan is playing for keeps! To think that before young boys and girls can even begin to make plans for their future, that future is practically ruined through intemperance. Parents especially need to be on guard and do everything we can to protect our children, God's children, from the evil devices of Satan.

A report in *The Lancet (1998;352:1433-1437)* revealed that the recreational drug 'ecstacy' was linked to brain damage in humans.

The Journal of the National Cancer Institute (1998;90:1198-1205) reports that smoking marijuana and cocaine can cause precancerous changes in the bronchial epithelium, the cells that line the airways to the lungs. "For the first time, our investigations show that tobacco is not the only smoked substance that sets in motion the molecular events that can lead to lung cancer."

What can be done? In the area of diet, an interesting experiment on laboratory rats is reported by Dr. Agatha Thrash in *Nature's Banquet p.112-113*. It sheds light on where many parents are failing. "Several animal studies indicate that the taste for 10% alcohol is easily controlled by the diet fed to them. In one experiment, rats were fed a diet typical of many Americans. When the rats were given the choice of water or 10% alcohol, they chose to drink **5 times** more alcohol solution than a paired group of rats fed a milk-vegetable diet.

"After stabilizing the diet for 10 weeks, the rats on the popular U.S. diet were consuming an average of over 40 ml. of 10% alcohol per 100 gm. body weight per week. They were then switched to the milk-vegetable diet. Within one week, the alcohol consumption had decreased to less than 5 ml., instead of 40 ml. previously consumed. In three weeks, the rats had almost completely stopped drinking alcohol.

Then the popular U.S. diet was resumed. Within four weeks,

thcy wcrc back up to 40 ml. On certain diets, the alcohol consumption could be doubled by simply adding coffee, and quadrupled when both coffee and spices were added."

The following chart show the results of one of these studies.

RELATIONSHIP BETWEEN DIET AND ALCOHOL USE IN LABORATORY ANIMALS!		
Rats eating foods below used alcohol as 52% of fluids	Rats eating diet below used alcohol as 18% of fluids	Rats on foods below used alcohol as 2.7% of fluids
Sweet rolls Doughnuts Hot Dogs Mustard Pickle Relish Spaghetti & Meatballs French Bread Apple Pie Green Beans Chopped Salad Chocolate Cake Candy Bar Cookie Coffee & Cake Eleven common spices	Standard Commercial Laboratory Chow Diet	Milk-Vegetable diet

Once again we see that the closer we follow God's original plan, the greater the blessings.

TOBACCO

One of the most pernicious habits by which an individual can he enslaved is the tobacco habit. It is one of Satan's most

61

effective inventions to shorten the life of God's people. For many years, tobacco use was thought to be beneficial, but with the Surgeon General's report in the sixties, tobacco was identified as the primary cause of many premature deaths in the U.S. and around the world. The evidence supporting this fact is overwhelming and cannot be ignored. Smoking may be associated with age-related hearing loss. Those who smoked had a 70% greater risk of hearing loss than nonsmokers. Smoking suppresses the body's ability to repair damage to blood vessels, leading to circulatory problems of all types. *(The Journal of the American Medical Association, 1998;279:1715-1719).*

Smoking is the primary risk factor in the development of lung cancer. It is more of a risk factor than is radon, a naturally occurring, odorless gas emitted by soil, water, building materials, and natural gas sources. Radon is believed to be the cause of between 7,000 and 30,000 deaths annually. *(American Journal of Public Health 1998;88811-812).*

Recent studies revealed an association between maternal smoking and attention-deficit hyperactivity disorder, ADHD. *(Archives of Disease in Childhood 1998; 79:207-212).* Maternal smoking is related to underweight newborns, a higher rate of perinatal morbidity and mortality, and even Sudden Infant Death Syndrome (SIDS). Maternal smoking also causes persistent deficits in learning and behavior. *(Journal of Pharmacology & Experimental Therapeutics 2853:931-945, June 1998).*

There was an increase incidence of kidney cancer in laboratory rats when exposed to tobacco smoke as reported in the Journal of the National Cancer Institute, November 1998 issue.

A study given by Christine Williams at the 71st annual American Heart Association meeting in Dallas, TX, 1998, revealed that "as parents do, so do the children." Children whose mothers smoked were six times more likely to smoke than children of nonsmoking parents. Another study by Dr. Merrill F. Elias of the University of Maine-Orono, given at the same meeting related smoking to a decrease in cognitive functioning or learning ability of children.

Another interesting fact concerning maternal and parental smoking is based on data compiled between 1988 and 1994. It included reports about household and maternal smoking during pregnancy. The researchers estimated that second-hand smoke was responsible for between 40 and 60 percent of all cases of asthma, bronchitis, and wheezing among young children. It does not take an Einstein to realize that smoking causes health problems among those that smoke and those who live with smokers.

Dr. John Wiencke of the University of California at San Francisco, reported in the April issue of the Journal of the National Cancer Institute that smoking in teenagers causes DNA changes that are linked to cancer. "Early age smoking, during a time of rapid lung growth and development, may induce long-lasting physiologic changes that impair the removal of damaged bases of the DNA." *(Journal of the National Cancer Institute 1999;91:578-579, 614-619)*

Secondhand smoke is as detrimental to those exposed to it, as smoking is to the smoker. In a report by the National Cancer Institute, not only lung cancer, but heart disease, nasal sinus cancer, Sudden Infant Death Syndrome and other diseases were associated with secondhand smoke. As stated earlier, middle ear infections, asthma, bronchitis and pneumonia in children have been linked to secondhand smoke. The administrator of the Environmental Protection Agency, Carol Browner says, "We again call on all parents to protect their children from exposure to secondhand cigarette smoke whenever possible." *(Reuters Health, New York, NY. , Nov. 23, 1999).* The recent banning of smoking in public buildings is long overdue. I am grateful to God for the recent changes in the public's attitude about smoking.

"Doc, I'd like to quit. But how can I?" Don't be discouraged, there are many successful programs to help you overcome the tobacco addiction. Participating in one of these programs like the American Cancer Society's program or "The Five-Day Plan" sponsored by the Seventh-day Adventist Church, may do the trick. But if you'd like to try it on your own, just comply with the simple guidelines below and I'm sure that, with God's blessings, you will be *"more than (a) conqueror through Him that loved us." (Rom. 8:37)* You will then be free from one of the most addicting substances known to man.

CONQUERING THE TOBACCO HABIT/ADDICTION

1. **Stop all caffeinated beverages!** (Coffee, soft drinks, tea, and chocolate.) Caffeine is chemically related to nicotine. Stopping caffeine before stopping tobacco will make the process much easier. Give yourself at least two weeks off caffeine before you stop the tobacco, unless you are participating in one of the smoking cessation programs. (White willow bark or Tylenol may be used to alleviate the caffeine withdrawal headaches, if they occur.)

2. **Drink at least 8 glasses of water every day!** Water will help eliminate nicotine from the body through the kidneys.
3. **Drink plenty of fruit juice!** Fruit juice also helps to eliminate nicotine. Make sure that the juices are sugar-free and 100% fruit juice.

4. **Do not use artificial sweeteners.** Some believe they act as a stimulant leading to tobacco use.

5. **You MUST NOT drink any alcoholic beverages!** This will definitely sabotage your program.

6. **Set a "stop date" and "talk it up."** Let everyone know that you are quitting the use of tobacco and try to get as much support as possible.

7. **Remember to** ASK GOD FOR HIS HELP! He has promised success, if you follow His program. Please read **Philippians 4:13, 19.**

8. **Promise to thank God and give Him the glory when**

65

you are successful! Also promise to direct others to Him, when asked how you quit this vile habit/addition.

Clinical Case #1: A 54-year-old Black female has a 20-year history of smoking one pack per day. She had been told to stop by her primary care physician but was unable to so. She started the BEST WAY program with the suggestions listed above for smoking cessation, and by God's grace she was tobacco free in two weeks, with "no desire" to smoke. She was amazed that it was "so easy!" *"Take my yoke upon you and learn of me, for my yoke is easy and my burden is light." (Matthew 11:30)*

Clinical Case #2: A 50-year-old Black female who heard the practical steps above while listening to our weekly radio broadcast came into the office with the testimony that she had stopped the use of tobacco after smoking for over 20 years. She was very thankful because she had attempted to quit many times without success.

I pray that this practical and simple program will help you or a loved one, as it has hundreds of others over the past 15 years, to be FREE AT LAST! MAY GOD BLESS.

WATER

"And he said unto me, It is done. I am Alpha and Omega, the beginning and the end. I will give unto him that is athirst of the fountain of the water of life freely." Revelation 21:6

"In health and in sickness, pure water is one of heaven's choicest blessings. Its proper use promotes health. It is the beverage which God provided to quench the thirst of animals and man. Drunk freely, it helps to supply the necessities of the system and assists nature to resist disease. The external application of water is one of the easiest and most satisfactory ways of regulating the circulation of the blood. A cold or cool bath is an excellent tonic. Warm baths open the pores and thus aid in the elimination of impurities. Both warm and neutral bath soothe the nerves and equalize the circulation." (White, E.G. Ministry of Healing p.237.001)

"Water is the universal medium in which all of the complex metabolic processes of life take place. Water is the largest single constituent of living cells, life itself depends upon a constant source of and utilization of water in the body." *(Kimber, Diana, et al. Anatomy and Physiology, 15th. Ed. New York: The MacMillan Co., 1966, p.665)* Water is essential for life and health.

Water comprises 50-60% of your body weight. In the above text we see our Creator offers us the *"water of life."* Christ says He is the *"Living Water,"* and anyone who comes to Him will never thirst again. *(See John 4:13, 14.)* But Satan has perverted our appetites, so that we prefer almost anything to water. I remember growing up in Daytona Beach, Florida where the water was not very palatable, in fact it was horrible.☺ I recall going days without drinking even one glass of water; though I did drink large quantities of orange juice, soft drinks and koolaid. I just did not like water. When I heard the analogy of Jesus likening Himself to water, I probably would not have wanted Him either, if my parents had not reared me to love and respect Him. But when I became extremely thirsty, water was the only beverage that would quench my thirst. And isn't it the same today! Jesus, the Living Water, is the only One that can quench the thirst of our souls.

Many patients and seminar attendees function as I once did and do not drink adequate water. This is the one beverage you should get an adequate supply of on a daily basis. You need at least 6-8 eight oz. glasses each day. Most are not aware that you need the same amount of water in the winter as you do in the summer. During the winter we sweat less but have an increase in the insensible water lost through the skin, due to winter's low humidity. Consequently our lips chap and our skin dries out and itches tremendously.

A survey conducted by the Nutrition Information Center at the New York Hospital-Cornell Medical Center observed that most Americans were getting only a third of the water they needed for optimal hydration. Two out of three knew they should drink eight, 8 oz. glasses of water daily. But only 21% drank the recommended amount. Thirty-five percent drank three or fewer glasses per day and 9% drank no water at all. Some of the survey respondents were actually drinking themselves into dehydration by consuming water-depleting beverages like caffeine and alcohol.

Water is important in the:

- regulation of your body temperature
- prevention and treatment of urinary tract infections
- prevention of kidney stones
- prevention and treatment of gouty arthritis.
- prevention and treatment of constipation
- prevention of headaches
- prevention and treatment of respiratory infections
- cleansing the body when externally applied
- prevention and treatment of dehydration
- prevention of keratoconjunctivitis sicca, or dry eyes
- proper function of every cell in the body
- prevention and treatment of dry and itchy skin
- prevention of myocardial infarctions, heart attacks

In a recent interview, Dr. Jeremy Matchett, a pharmacy professor and associate dean of the University of Kansas School of Pharmacy confirmed that water ingestion is crucial in the treatment of colds and flu. He states that when it comes to whether you should "feed a cold and starve a fever," the best approach is to "drown both of them."☺ In fact, I have found through personal experience, that using a vaporizer or humidifier in the winter, is one of the best measures that can be used in preventing sore throats, colds, and sinus infections.

In a study of over 34,000 Seventh-day Adventists, Jacqueline Chan, Ph.D., reported that drinking at least five glasses of water each day was associated with a significant decrease in the risk of fatal heart attacks. This was among persons without a history of heart disease, stroke or diabetes. The study was reported at the 20th Congress of the European Society of Cardiology.

Her colleague, Dr. Synnove F. Knutsen, reported that among

69

those with a history of heart disease, stroke or diabetes, drinking a minimum of five glasses of water each day, lowered the risk of fatal strokes. Both were thought to be due to a decrease in the blood viscosity or thickness. This decreases the possibility of blood clotting. Optimal hydration comes by drinking 6-8 glasses of water each day.

"Compared with those who drank less than two glasses of water a day, men who drank five or more glasses had a 51% decreased risk of fatal coronary heart disease; women who drank five or more glasses had a 35% lower risk of fatal heart attacks. Those who drank five or more glasses of water a day had a 44% decreased risk of fatal stroke, compared with those who drank two or fewer glasses, after adjusting for traditional risk factors." *(Internal Medicine News 31[19]six, October 1, 1998)*

Another study reported in the journal *Circulation, 1998;97:1467-1473* identified blood viscosity as a risk factor for heart disease. So, please, drink water freely, for your health.

But you may be saying, "My water is so bad, with all those chemicals, and pollutants. Just what is the best type of water to drink?" I am asked that question at practically every seminar in which I participate. My 'patented' answer is a question, "what type do you like?" They then give me their preference of either distilled, spring, mineral or some other type. I answer; "then that is the best water for you!"☺ In fact, the water supply in the United States is actually quite safe, with few disease causing bacteria or chemicals present. Most problems are with the esthetics or taste of the water. If the taste of the water in your area is a problem, just buy a charcoal filter that fits on the faucet or the refrigerator's water dispenser. And, abracadabra, good tasting water.☺

From a scientific basis, the purest water is distilled. There are no solid substances in distilled water. It is also essentially sodium-free. It is flat tasting because the minerals have been removed. The minerals give water its satisfying taste.

"Mineral water" comes from springs and contains those minerals that are present in that locality. The bottled water industry is essentially unregulated, therefore no specific standards exist which tells the consumer what is in the water except for the sodium content. It has been reported, though I am not sure of its accuracy, that some bottled water is just water from the tap placed in bottles. *(The Wellness Encyclopedia, University of California, Berkeley p.492-3, Houghton Mifflin Company, 1991)*

So what type of water do I drink? TAP, run through a charcoal filter, and it is good. I'm not going to pay for what I can get free, no way!☺ **So please,** drink enough water, and take the "Water of Life" freely every day.

HYDROTHERAPY

Water can also be applied externally in the prevention and treatment of virtually all diseases known to man. This is termed hydrotherapy, the use of water in the prevention and treatment of disease and illness. Jesus and the prophet Elisha used hydrotherapy in the healing of the sick during their ministries. Naaman the leper was told to wash in the Jordan river seven times by Elisha. *(See 2 Kings 5:1-14)* The blind man was healed by Jesus when Jesus put clay on his eyes and then had him wash in the pool of Siloam *(See John 9:1-7)*. Both are Biblical examples of this marvelous treatment modality.

Water is a versatile substance created by God for the benefit of man, animals and plants. It is useful in each of its physical states. It is the only substance found in nature in the solid, liquid, and gaseous state. God created water for your benefit and you should become familiar with its uses.

The reason water is such an excellent substance to use in the treatment of disease is because of its ability to absorb heat, which is called *specific heat*. "A pound of water would communicate thirty times as much heat to the body as a pound of mercury at the same temperature." *(Thomas, Charles S., Water Seminar p.100:9, School of Health, Loma Linda University, 1977)* Heat causes an increase in the metabolism of all cells of the body.

Remember the Bible states that, *"the life of the flesh is in the blood" (Lev. 17:11)*. To have perfect health, the blood supply or circulation must be perfect. Water can be used to manipulate the circulation of the blood in the body. Heat applied to an area caused an increase in the blood flow to that area. This is the result of the relaxing effect or dilation of the smooth muscles in the blood vessels.

Cold water rapidly absorbs heat when it comes in contact with other objects. When placed on the skin, it quickly cools the area. The effect of which is blood vessel constriction. This results in a decrease in the blood flow to that area. Thus, we can easily manipulate the flow of blood in the body.

Water's physiological effects can be placed in two categories and are determined by the temperature of the water applied. The intrinsic or direct effect is one category and the reaction is the other category. The reaction is made up of a series of physiologic changes initiated by the body in an effort to counteract the intrinsic effect of the hot or cold water. The reaction is seen with the prolonged application of cold or heat.

Cold applied for a prolonged period of time causes vasoconstriction, and a slowing down of the metabolism in the area. This is its **intrinsic effect**. When applied to a large part of the body for a long period, cold can cause a decrease in respiration, a slowing of the pulse, and a decrease or cessation of digestion. Tactile sensations are blunted and with time the body temperature is lowered. Examples of these effects are seen when your fingers are exposed to cold temperatures and become numb, or when your face is exposed to the cold for a prolonged period affecting your speech. These are the intrinsic or direct effects of the cold itself.

The **reaction** occurs when the body begins to counteract the intrinsic effects of the cold in its attempts to return the temperature to normal. Vasodilation leads to an increase in

the blood flow to the affected area increasing the body

temperature. The reaction has the opposite physiologic effect of the intrinsic action. When generalized cold is applied, the heart rate, the respiratory rate, and the digestive processes all increase as a **reaction** to the cold. Many of the most important and beneficial results of hydrotherapy are due to the reaction. "It is this arousing of the body to aid in its own recuperation and healing that characterizes natural or physiological therapy." *(Thomas, Charles S., Water Seminar p.100:13, School of Health, Loma Linda University, 1977)*

The reaction consists of three phases:
1. A thermic phase (example: in **response** to cold, the body produces more heat.)
2. A circulatory phase (example: in **response** to cold the skin becomes reddened due to an increase in the blood flow to the area.)
3. A nervous phase (example: in **response** to cold the nerves begin to tingle and there is a feeling of renewed energy, caused by the stimulation of nervous activity.)

These three phases make up the **reaction**. They are not independent of each other but occur simultaneously. It is the circulatory phase, manifested by the changes in the skin color, that lets you know that the reaction is complete.

Whether the intrinsic effect predominates over the reaction, depends upon the intensity and duration of the intrinsic effect. This is seen when an ice bag is placed on a sprained ankle. The prolonged and intense application of cold causes suppression of metabolism and vasoconstriction leading to a decrease in inflammation and swelling. This reduces tissue damage and leads to a more rapid recovery from the sprain.

The various temperatures that are important when using hydrotherapy are below.

♦	Very hot	104°F and above
♦	Hot	100-103°F
♦	Warm (neutral 94-97)	92-100°F
♦	Tepid	80-92°F
♦	Cool	70-80°F
♦	Cold	55-70°F
♦	Very cold	32-55°F

The physiologic effects of the different temperatures are as follows:

1. *Short cold & contrast procedures* (hot followed by cold) are stimulants causing a tonic effect.
2. *Prolonged cold* is a depressant. It also has an antipyretic (fever reducing) and decongestant effect. It causes vasoconstriction.
3. *Mild heat* acts as a sedative and causes relaxation.
4. *Moderate heat* causes perspiration because of peripheral vasodilation leading to sweating, and a moderate rise in body temperature.
5. *Marked heat* is a stimulant and causes an increase in metabolism and circulation.

In my home and at work, we use hydrotherapy for the common illnesses that confront us. In the office, hydrotherapy is recommended for every patient. These simple treatments produce an effect that is beneficial to the body because of its affect on the circulatory, endocrine, nervous, muscular, digestive, and immune systems.

Now for some important guidelines when giving hydrotherapy treatments.

IMPORTANT FACTORS WHEN GIVING HYDROTHERAPY TREATMENTS

A. The Place where the treatment is given must be:
1. Warm
2. Free of drafts
3. Free of bright light in the patient's eyes
4. Protected from water damage, (furniture, rugs, bedding, etc.)
5. Cleaned after the treatment
B. The Treatment itself:
1. Think and plan ahead.
2. Assemble all necessary articles before starting and prepare the treatment area.
3. Spread a drape sheet over the table to prevent chilling of the patient.
4. Stay with the patient or be within easy calling distance.
5. Don't talk too much.
6. Observe the physiologic reaction to the treatment.
7. Make any changes in the treatment rapidly.
C. The Patient:
1. Must be warm before the treatment begins. (You may use a hot foot bath, a warm drink of herb tea or more covers.)
2. Must be undress for practically all treatments.
3. You must explain the procedure to the patient; what you will be doing and what effect it should have. **DO NOT SURPRISE THE PATIENT**, especially with cold applications. *(Thomas,*

Charles S., Water Seminar p.1000:7, School of Health, Loma Linda University, 1977)

a. When using a heating treatment use a cold compress to the head and neck.
b. Follow modesty and do not unnecessarily expose the patient. (Uncover only the part under immediate treatment.)
c. Dry the area thoroughly after the treatment.
d. Keep the patient as comfortable as possible at all times.
e. Keep the patient relaxed.
f. Demand that the patient rest after the treatment.
g. Avoid chilling!
h. No sweating should be present when the patient dresses. (A state of heat conservation.)

Now that you have a little background in the effect of different temperatures of water on the body and also a few guidelines on giving hydrotherapy treatment, you are ready to begin your quest of "healing the sick and stamping out disease."☺ These specific treatments can be done at home with little, if any, outlay of finances.

HOT TUB BATH

When doing this treatment you should have someone available to help you if needed.

Articles needed:
1. Three bath towels
2. Two wash cloths
3. A mouth thermometer
4. A basin of cool water
5. Ice Bag

Procedure:
1. Fill tub 2/3 full of hot water (104-105°F)
2. Put a folded towel behind the head for comfort.
3. Cover exposed body parts with a towel.
4. Keep the head cool with a compress or the ice bag.
5. The duration of the treatment should be 10-15 minutes in adults and 3-5 minutes in children.
6. Cool the water to 98° for 3-5 minutes before standing to avoid dizziness and fainting then take a cool shower. This closes the pores of the skin preventing excessive heat loss and the tendency to chill.
7. Dry off briskly and then rest for 30-60 minutes.

Indications for this treatment:
Colds, flu, arthritis, poor circulation, muscle stiffness, and congestion of internal organs.

Contraindications for this treatment:
Heart or valvular diseases (heart attacks, mitral valve prolapse, angina pectoris), cancer, diabetes, circulation problems, and high blood pressure.

Precautions:
Senior citizens, frail or weak persons should not use this treatment. If dizziness or faintness occurs, **STOP AT ONCE AND COOL THE PERSON.**

HEATING COMPRESS

Articles needed:
1. Cotton cloth folded double, wide enough to cover the area being treated.
2. A piece of flannel or wool, single or double, long enough to wrap around the area and at least 2 inches wider than the cotton cloth.
3. Safety pins.

Procedure:
1. Wet the cotton cloth in cold water, wring it out (should be wet and cold but not drippy), apply around the affected area.
2. Cover the cotton cloth well with the wool or flannel. It should fit snugly but not too tightly.
3. Pin securely and leave on for several hours or overnight. The body will cause the compress to warm up.
4. If the compress does not heat up in 10-15 minutes dress warmer and put feet in hot water (unless you are diabetic or have circulatory problems.)
5. After removing the compress, immediately rub the area with a cold cloth and then dry briskly.

Indications for this treatment:
Sore throat, laryngitis, chronic rheumatic joint conditions, painful joints, chest congestions, and bronchitis.

When using the heating compress on the chest for congestion, you should apply a tee shirt without sleeves wrung out in cold water and cover it with a flannel top. Keep on overnight, then rub the chest with a cool cloth and dry off briskly.

CONTRAST BATHS OR SOAKS

Articles Needed:
1. Two containers large enough to cover affected area.
2. Bath towels

Procedure:
1. Place affected area in the hot water (between 105-110° F) for 3 minutes. Test the water with your elbow if you do not have a thermometer. **WARNING: The temperature should not be above 105° if you have diabetes or circulatory problems in the feet or legs.**
2. Then place affected area in the very cold water for thirty seconds. (Use ice in the water unless you have diabetes or circulatory problems.)
3. Change from one temperature to another for 3 cycles, ending in cold water.
4. Dry area briskly with a towel.

Indications for this treatment:
Infections, cellullitis, edema, lymphagitis, poor circulation, arthritis, or weak feet. Ankle, foot or hand sprains after 24-48 hours of ice only.

Contraindications for this treatment:
Cancer, DIABETES, and peripheral vascular diseases.

Precautions:
Do not use this treatment if you have diabetes or blood vessel diseases like atherosclerosis. For these conditions use only warm and cool water for the contrast baths.

CONTRAST SHOWERS

Purpose or effects: This is good treatment for many conditions. It is stimulating in nature. The intrinsic effect of heat causes an increase in the metabolic rate and blood vessels dilation. Cold by contrast causes blood vessels to constrict. This treatment acts as a vascular gymnastic. The short cold also acts as a stimulant.

Procedure:
1. Take a shower increasing temperature as tolerated.
2. Hold that temperature for 3 minutes.
3. Lower the temperature by turning the hot water down to the lowest tolerated temperature; hold for 30 seconds.
4. Repeat contrast for 2-3 cycles.
5. Complete the treatment with a brisk towel rub.
6. Rest for 20-30 minutes prior to resuming regular activities.

Indications for this treatment:
1. Hypertension - leads to improved blood vessels compliance
2. As a vigorous tonic of drowsiness.
3. To stimulate the metabolism.
4. To stimulate the immune system.
5. When debilitated by a sedentary lifestyle.

Contraindications for this treatment:
A nervousness, irritable, or excited state of mind.

NEUTRAL TUB BATH

Purposes or Effects:
1   To relax the body
2.   To sedate the nervous system
3.   To provide sedation for the patient with diseases of the heart and blood vessels who cannot tolerate hot and cold treatments.

Procedure:
1.   Get in the tub with an air pillow or folded towel behind the head.
2.   Cover the exposed parts of the body with a towel or the tub with a sheet.
3.   Instruct the patient to lie quietly and relax. Use a cold compress to the forehead as needed to keep the head cool.
4.   Maintain a constant water temperature.
5.   The duration of the treatment: 15 minutes to 4 hours.
6.   After the treatment, dry off quickly but avoid unnecessary rubbing. Lie down and rest for 30-60 minutes.

Indications for this treatment:
1.   Central nervous system exhaustion
2.   Insomnia
3.   Nervous irritability

Important Considerations:
1.   The temperature will vary with the condition of the patient, season of the year, and the temperature of the room.
2.   The patient should be warm before taking a neutral bath.
3.   If the patient is in the bath longer than 4 hours, lubricate the skin with a lanolin cream.

STEAM INHALATION

Purposes and Effects:
1. To relieve inflammation & congestion of the sinuses.
2. To relieve throat irritation.
3. To loosen secretions and stimulate the discharge of mucous from the throat, lungs, and sinuses.
4. To relax muscles and relieve coughing.
5. To keep mucous membranes from excessive drying.

Procedure:
1. Heat water to the boiling point in a kettle.
2. Add medication (Eucalyptus, pine oil) if desired.
3. Place a towel over the head and catch the steam with the towel. If the person is in bed use an umbrella.
4. Breathe slowly and deeply.
5. Continue treatment for 30-60 minutes, repeat 2-3 times a day as needed.

Indications for this treatment:
1. Coughing.
2. Chest congestion.
3. Throat irritation
4. Dry throat & sinuses.
5. Infection in the sinuses or upper respiratory tract.

Contraindications for this treatment:
1. Very young children or very old adults.

These are just a few of the many hydrotherapy treatments that can be done in the home to help prevent illnesses or treat illnesses. While living in New York, my wife and two young daughters came down with the flu. They looked so pitiful laid out on the couch. I could not afford to be sick, so I gave myself the hot tub bath treatment every night until they had recovered. Good common sense like, refraining from kissing my wife until she had fully recuperated, was exercised. I DID NOT CATCH THE FLU. I'm sure that the hydrotherapy treatments were blessed of God, and helped in the prevention of this illness.

But remember, even though these remedies are based upon sound physiologic principles, God is the one who heals. When you pray before the treatment you will be amazed to see God answer in such a marked manner.

There are other hydrotherapy treatments that are beneficial. If you want to become more familiar with them or would like a more in-depth source of information on hydrotherapy, please consult one of the following books:

1. **Home Remedies**, by Drs. Agatha and Calvin Thrash, Uchee Pines Institute, Seale, AL 36875
2. **Simple Remedies for the Home**, by Clarence W. Dail, M.D. and Charles S. Thomas, Ph.D., Teach Services, Brushton, New York.

FEVER

Fever is one of the most misunderstood operations of the human body. It is looked upon with dread and fear by many, when in fact, it is of great benefit to your body. It helps you in recovering from illnesses that are due to infections.

Fever is defined as an elevation of your body temperature above normal. The normal body temperature is 98.6°F in most people. Anything above this is termed a fever. Many get very nervous if the temperature gets above 98.6°F, but fever is your friend and not your foe! It is a God ordained response of your body to invasions by virulent organisms and other harmful agents. Causes of fever include:

1. Infections (viral, bacterial, fungi, protozoan, ect.)
2. Cancers, especially lymphomas.
3. Tissue death such as chemical or mechanical injuries, myocardial infarction, or pulmonary emboli.
4. Foreign proteins in the blood (lactation, venomous bites, ect.)
5. Dehydration
6. Increased thyroid activity.
7. Muscular or chemical activity.

(Thrash, A. and Thrash, C.; Home Remedies, p.23)

The beneficial effects of fever on the body are many and include:

1) An increase in the white blood cells in the circulation (the cells responsible for fighting infections and cancer).
2) An increase in interferon, a substance produced in the body that acts to destroy all viruses. It inhibits cancer causing viruses and directly inhibits tumor cell

85

growth.

3) Enhances the removal of wastes from the blood.
4) An increase in the blood flow to the skin where specific white blood cells, fixed macrophages, purify the blood and adds chemicals that make germs more capable of being destroyed. (Ibid.)

You have nothing to fear unless the body temperature gets above 102°F. If this should occur, you should begin measures to reduce the temperature to or near normal. But fevers below 102°F are doing you good, not harm!

What should you do if you or one of your family members runs a fever? Different temperatures require different measures. If the temperature is between 99-103°, you should do a hot tub bath with a cold compress or ice pack to the head. This brings the blood to the skin where the heat can be released. Finish this with a cool shower and dry off briskly with a towel. This principle was used by my mother on each of her nine children and also on my father. (They saved the best for last. Guess who is the youngest? That's right! Me.☺) She would pile blankets on us when we had a fever. I would say to myself, "I'm already hot, why am I under all these blankets?" This caused us to perspire which is the way the body dissipates heat. Thus the temperature was decreased and the fever alleviated.

So you have nothing to fear when it comes to fevers. It's one of the body's ways of keeping infections from becoming more serious.

AIR

"And the Lord God formed man of the dust of the ground, and breathed into his nostrils the breath of life; and man became a living soul." (Gen. 2:7)

The breath of life breathed into man was the pure air formulated by God for His creation. Every plant, animal, and human being is dependent upon air for survival. Man can live weeks without food, days without water, but only minutes without air.

The primary gas needed by man and animal is oxygen. Every cell in the body is dependent upon it for survival. The interdependence of man and his environment is clearly seen by the fact that man breathes in oxygen and exhales carbon dioxide. Plants use this carbon dioxide for growth, and produce oxygen as a byproduct. Oxygen enters the body through the lungs. It is carried by the hemoglobin in red blood cells to every cell in the body. I'm reminded of the statement that says, *"In order to have good blood, we must breathe well. Full deep inspirations of pure air, which fill the lungs with oxygen, purify the blood. They impart to it a bright color, and send it, a life-giving current, to every part of the body. Good respirations soothe the nerves; it stimulates the appetite and renders digestion more perfect; it induces sound, refreshing sleep ...[if] an insufficient supply of oxygen is received, the blood moves sluggishly. The waste, poisonous matter, which should be thrown off in the exhalations from the lungs, is retained, and the blood becomes impure. Not only the lungs, but the stomach, liver, and brain are affected. The skin becomes sallow, digestion is retarded; the heart is depressed; the brain is clouded; the thoughts are confused; gloom settles upon the spirits; the whole system becomes depressed and inactive, and peculiarly susceptible to disease." (White, E. G., Ministry of Healing, p.237, 272).*

When breathing normally, you use only about 1/10 to 1/20 of your lung capacity. No wonder you become so easily irritated and sluggish of thought. Exercise, causes deeper breathing and is very healthful to the body. You need to take three deep breaths, three times each day to adequately fill the lungs. If we are irritable, deep breathing is very soothing to the nerves.

In some of our major cities, air pollution is a big problem. With the rapid growth and construction of more and more buildings, and the destruction of even more trees and plants; the air is not ideal in any area of our country. But our Savior knows all these things, and He knows you can only do the best you can. Those things that are out of your control, you should not worry about. But leave them in the hands of your Savior Jesus Christ. However, you must do what you can. Below, you will find practical aids to improve your health.

1. Live, as far as possible, in an unpolluted environment.
2. Maintain correct posture while standing and sitting in order to breathe correctly.
3. Do not restrict the free movement of the abdominal and chest muscles by wearing clothes like girdles, tight jeans, etc., that compress these areas.
4. Develop the habit of taking at least three deep breaths, three times each day.
5. Sleep with your windows cracked or open, unless your property or life might be threatened by doing so.
   (Adapted from Natures Banquet by Living Springs Retreat, p.101.)

YIELDING TRUST IN GOD'S POWER

> *"Trust in the Lord with all your heart, and lean not unto your own understanding." (Prov.3:5). "Trust in Him at all times; ye people, pour out your heart before Him; God is a refuge for us."(Ps 62:8). "What time I am afraid, I will trust in thee." (Ps 56:3)*

I saved the best for last! We all trust someone or something, it is a part of our nature. When you take a cab, you trust the driver to take you to your destination, even though you do not know him. You also trust the pilots of the aircrafts to fly it safely to your desired destination. Trust is an inherent quality that God placed in each of us. Notice how a small child will jump from heights which are gigantic in his eyes into his or her father's arms. Our Father, our Creator and Saviour, asked us to trust in Him.

You can trust God because He is trustworthy. I know you have experienced times in your life, as I have; when you didn't know how you were going to make it! Maybe financial problems stalked you, or maybe social or family difficulties plagued you. You soon exhausted all of your options and had nowhere or no one else to turn but to Jesus, and He came through like He always does.

These experiences are given that you and I might have more faith in Him. *"For without faith it is impossible to please Him."* *(Heb.11:6)* But is this a blind faith lacking scientific evidence? I say that experience is the best teacher. If I know by experience what God has done for me, I don't need anything more. I have tasted and have seen, *"that the Lord is good." (Ps 34:8)*

But if scientific evidence helps to increase your faith, some interesting studies showing the part that faith plays in health and healing have recently been published.

Mitch Krucoff, M.D., a cardiologist, and Suzanne Crater a nurse practitioner, performed one such study at the Durham Veterans Affairs Medical Center in North Carolina. Cardiac patients were randomly divided into five treatment groups of 30 patients each. All patients received traditional medical therapies. Each participant's name in one of the groups was sent to prayer circles around the world. Neither the patients nor the investigator knew which group was being prayed for. This is what we term a "double blind" study. All of the patients went through an invasive procedure which involved threading a catheter through arteries into the heart to collect images or to clear clogged arteries. The group receiving prayer during their hospital stay did 50% to 100% better than those who did not. *(Reported in Reuters Health, Dec. 24, 1998)*

Other studies show that having strong religious convictions are associated with a longer life expectancy, lower blood pressure, and a stronger immune system. *"My son, forget not my law; but let thine heart keep my commandments: For length of days, and long life, and peace, shall they add to thee." (Proverbs 3:1,2)*

In the *American Journal of Public Health 1998; 88:1469-1475*, it was reported that senior citizens who attended church services live longer than those who do not. Younger adults who participate in religious activities tend to have lower blood pressures, lower rates of heart disease, fewer, symptoms of depression, and lower death rates than those who did not participate.

In Novato, California, Drs. Douglas Oman and Dwayne Reed followed 2,000 volunteers ages 55 and older for five years. They completed a questionnaire to access their health habits, mental health, and their level of social support. They were also questioned regarding their religious service attendance. Health records were reviewed and tests to measure physical functioning were administered. After five years, those who attended religious services were 24% less likely to have died than those that did not. This was after other factors were taken into consideration including, age, sex, health, mental health status, and level of social support. Even among those with the highest levels of social support, religious involvement was still associated with an even lower risk of death.

In my practice, I always offer to have prayer for my patients. Over the past 20 years, I have witnessed the miracle working power of God, in answer to prayer. I praise God for answered prayers!

Chapter 5

MODERN MEDICINE AND NATURAL HEALING

"But thou, O Daniel, shut up the words, and seal the book, even to the time of the end: many shall run to and fro, and knowledge shall be increased." Daniel 12:4

In our world today, we have reached a state of affairs where anything and everything goes. In the area of health, this too, is the case. Because of the distrust that many have in modern medicine, there has been an abandonment of many time-honored techniques and procedures, for what is called an "all natural" approach. And while I am a traditionally trained physician, who uses natural methods of healing, I know that medical advances have prolonged the lives of millions the world over. Let's consider briefly some of these advances.

92

ANTIBIOTICS

Not many years ago, infectious diseases were the #1 cause of death. But with the advent of antibiotics in 1928, this has all changed. Today, very few people in this country die from rheumatic heart disease, which is a bacterial infection that can affect the heart valves and is caused by a group A streptococcus bacteria. The reason: the use of antibiotics. Pneumonia, once a feared and deadly illness, has for the most part, been tame to the point that very few deaths occur from this illness, when compared to the pre antibiotic era. Death rates from all infectious diseases have been greatly reduced since the introduction of antibiotics. Let God be praised for this wonderful discovery!

But now, the pendulum has swung to the other extreme! Antibiotics are being prescribed for even routine infections which the body's own defenses would eradicate if only given the chance. Most of these infections are viral in nature and antibiotics are of absolutely no benefit. Antibiotics do kill bacteria, but not viruses. Parents come to the physician's office literally demanding antibiotics for their child's cold. Doctors sometimes feel pressured, and prescribe antibiotics even though they know they will not help. It may even be somewhat detrimental for the patient to take them. But in an effort to satisfy and appease the parent or patient, the antibiotic is given. Because of this wholly unnecessary use of antibiotics, many resistant organisms are emerging, which "eat our antibiotics for lunch."

A typical example of this is seen when a mother comes into the office with her child, complaining of a sore throat. The child is not running a fever, but she does have a runny nose. The mucus is clear or white. The cough is productive of whitish phlegm and is associated with chest discomfort. She also has body aches. Diagnosis: This child has a viral upper respiratory infection for which antibiotics are of no benefit at all. But the mother demands an antibiotic, and instead of incurring her wrath, the physician gives her the prescription.

The psalmist, in *Psalms 139:14* says, *"I will praise thee; for I am fearfully and wonderfully made: marvelous are thy works; and that my soul knoweth right well."* If hygienic principles are followed and God's remedies used, there would be little need for antibiotics. Case in point; in the 37 years of the combined lives of my daughters, they have only taken one or two prescriptions of antibiotics between the two of them. We will discuss the natural treatment of common illnesses in chapter 8.

IMMUNIZATIONS

Immunizations have almost eradicated diseases like smallpox, mumps, measles, rubella, and tetanus. Many times I am asked the question, "Do you recommend that children get their baby shots?" I always answer, "My children are up-to-date on theirs!"☺ While there have been incidences when immunizations have caused serious harm to patients, these have been few and far between. I recommend that all children be immunized, unless there are medical reasons that would prohibit their administration.

Influenza vaccines are recommended for all adults over the age of 65 and for those with chronic diseases like diabetes, heart disease, hypertension, etc. If those who have been advised to have a flu shot would take it, then between 10,000 and 30,000 lives could be saved each year.

SURGERY

Surgical procedures have prolonged the lives of millions. Appendicitis, a very common condition, rarely causes death today because of the diagnostic and surgical advances that have been made. Coronary bypass surgery, once a novel procedure, is now being performed routinely and has extended the lives of hundreds of thousands. Significant suffering has been greatly reduced by the replacement of degenerated joints, removal of inflamed and infected gallbladders, removal of enlarged uteri and stones in the kidneys and gallbladders.

So do I, as a preventive lifestyle physician, recommend surgery for my patients? You best believe I do!☺ God was the first surgeon. He, of course, did not need a scalpel. The Bible states, *" And the LORD God caused a deep sleep to fall upon Adam, and he slept: and he took one of his ribs, and closed up the flesh instead thereof; And the rib, which the LORD God had taken from man, made he a woman, and brought her unto the man." (Genesis two: 21, 22)* Another example of the principle of surgery in the Word of God occurred when Jesus said, *"And if thy right hands offend thee, cut it off, and cast it from thee," (Matt. 5:30).* So if your gallbladder, appendix, or cataract offends thee, cut it out and cast it from thee.☺

DRUG MEDICATIONS

Multitudes of medications have been developed that lower blood pressure, blood sugar, cholesterol, and triglyceride levels. Others reduce or eliminate fevers, pains, aches, and other symptoms. Most have enhanced the quality of life and increased the life-expectancy. We should thank God for these advances. However, in the majority of cases, unless the individual changes their way of living, the problem will only return with vengeance. Christ, when He healed during His life on earth, often said, *"go, and sin no more." (John 8:11)* This teaches that when God works, and there is healing, you have the responsibility of living up to the light you have, in taking care of His temple, your body.

Great advances have been made in engendering a healthier and happier populous. But with the HMO's and manage care companies eroding the more personalized delivery of health care, many are searching for alternatives. Quality health care is deteriorating because many physicians are unable to spend time with their patients, due to the need to meet patient quotas. There is the pushing of one pill after another on the already, pill-saturated patient. Most patients know that this is not the best thing for them. Therefore patients are turning to "alternative modalities," some of which are questionable at best. I will discuss this in the next chapter of this book.

My greatest disenchantment with modern medicine is that we concentrate our efforts in treating patients when they get sick, with one pill or another, and do not properly educate them in how to live. We don't show them how to prevent illnesses through lifestyle changes and so we have patients on fifteen different medications. And God only knows what they are doing in that patient's body. We must put more emphasis, more money, and more efforts into prevention, because, **"an ounce of prevention is worth a TON of cure."**☺

RADIATION

What about radiation? This, I believe, is a rational medical treatment. Man has taken certain spectrums of light and intensified them. This provides for the destruction of tumor cells. Light is focused on the mass itself and causes very little serious damage to surrounding tissues and organs. Therefore if you are a candidate for radiation therapy, I would recommend you receive it, unless there are contraindications in your particular case.

CHEMOTHERAPY

Chemotherapy is a "horse of a different color." These are literal poisons. They are administered to treat different types of cancers, with the hope that they will kill more cancer cells than normal cells. They destroy bone marrow cells in many instances, and have a side-effect profile which strike fear in the hearts of all who read them. This approach I do not endorse except in very rare circumstances.

ROUTINE PHYSICAL EXAMINATIONS

I urge you get your regular physical examinations. Because **"what you don't know could kill you!"** We do know that the earlier a disease process is detected, the greater the chance for a cure. Most cancers are present for years before physical manifestations are seen. Routine screening examinations can detect them before they spread to the point where they are incurable, resulting in premature death; unless God works a miracle! The following table list the examinations that are recommended by the United States Preventive Services Task Force in their 1996 report.

SCREENING TEST	FREQUENCY
Blood Pressure	At least every 2 years
Breast examination	Annually after age 40
Hearing	Periodically ask older patients abut their hearing
Vision	Periodic screening with Snellen acuity testing
Cholesterol	Every 5 years
Pap Smear	Every 2 to 3 years
Stool occult blood	Annually after age 50
Mammography	Annually after age 50
Flexible sigmoidoscopy	Every 3 to 5 years after age 50
Counseling	Annually
Tetanus-diphtheria booster	Every 10-15 years
Influenza vaccine	Annually after age 65
Pneumococcal vaccine	Once after age 65
Digital rectal exam	Annually after age 40 years (after 35 in Blacks)
PSA (Prostate Specific Antigen)	No definite recommendations (I personally recommend this exam annually after age 55, and every 3 years after age 35.)

Therefore, it is imperative that you have annual physical examinations. It just may save your life!

God has blessed man with a vast amount of knowledge in the field of medicine and we should use all rational means to promote health and to cure disease. Most of these advances are beneficial, but when used as a means of controlling the symptoms and not addressing the cause, it's like "blowing in the wind."☺ Those habits that are responsible for the disease process, must be changed!

While we praise God for the knowledge He has given us in the treatment of disease, the true remedies, the **"BEST WAY,"** will never be out-of-date, regardless of medical advances. They must be an integral component of any program instituted for the prevention and treatment of disease.

CHAPTER 6

COUNTERFEIT REMEDIES?

> *" Therefore rejoice, ye heavens, and ye that dwell in them. Woe to the inhabiters of the earth and of the sea! for the devil is come down unto you, having great wrath, because he knoweth that he hath but a short time." "For there shall arise false Christs, and false prophets, and shall shew great signs and wonders; insomuch that, if it were possible, they shall deceive the very elect." (Revelations 12:12; Matthew 24:24)*

The above scriptures warn that in the end time, which is now, Satan will work to destroy and deceive God's people, even by performing miracles. He did this in the Garden of Eden when he came to the woman in the form of a serpent **(See Genesis 3)**. In Egypt, during the time of Moses, Satan once again worked miracles through the magicians of Pharaoh. He made what appeared to be snakes, from rods, and turned water red like blood, counterfeiting God's true miracles. He also made frogs appear from everywhere producing yet another counterfeit. **(See Genesis 7,8)**

During the life of Paul in the New Testament, we see several references pertaining to Satan's ability to perform supernatural feats. In *Acts 16:16* we read, *"And it came to pass, as we went to prayer, a certain damsel possessed with a spirit of divination met us, which brought her masters much gain by soothsaying (prophesying):"* Satan sought to undermine the confidence of the people in the message being preached by Paul. This was done through the workings of an evil spirit. Another incident that displays the miracle working power of Satan during the time of the New Testament church is here quoted: *"But there was a certain man, called Simon, which beforetime in the same city used sorcery, and bewitched the people of Samaria, giving out that himself was some great one: To whom they all gave heed, from the least to the greatest, saying, This man is the great power of God." (Acts: 9,10)* Therefore we can readily see that miracles, even undeniable ones, cannot form the basis of our beliefs.

"To the law and to the testimony, it they speak not according to this word, there is no light in them." (Isaiah 8:20) The Word of God is the standard by which all things must be measured. To discern whether something is true and from God, or is a counterfeit and from Satan, can only be determined by the unerring Word of God.

God's remedies, the **"BEST WAY,"** are found in His Word. But for every remedy of God, Satan has legions of counterfeits.

He does not counterfeit something that is not true. Even you would not try to counterfeit a $18.00 bill, would you? The story is told of a man who made a $18.00 bill and took it to the cashier of a grocery store and asked, "Can you please give me change for this $18.00 bill?" The cashier replied, "Sure! How do you want it? 2 nines, 3 sixes, or 6 threes?"☺

A counterfeit is something that closely resembles the original. And in the field of health there is no scarcity of counterfeits. How can you tell if a particular approach is one that should be avoided? Any technique, remedy, or treatment that leads us away from God or does not uplift Christ as the Great Physician, must be looked upon with suspicion. Their origin can also be used as an indicator of their legitimacy and safety. The statement of warning found below, may serve as a safeguard against the deceptions of the enemy.

"All who do not earnestly search the Scriptures and submit every desire and purpose of life to that unerring test, all who do not seek God in prayer for a knowledge of His will, will surely wander from the right path and fall under the deception of Satan.... His agents still claim to cure disease. They attribute their power to **electricity**, **magnetism** or the so-called '**sympathetic** remedies.' In truth, they are but channels for Satan's electric currents. By this means he cast his spell over the bodies and souls of men." *(E.G. White, Testimonies to the Church, Volume 5; p.192-193)*

The New Age movement has infiltrated every facet of society, including the area of health and wellness, and is captivating millions. Many sincere, honest, and loving people have embraced this "new teaching," which is not new, but is as old as time itself. Most are not aware of the origin of this philosophy and they accept it because "god" is mentioned, or because it works in many instances. Among its adherents, there is this feeling of togetherness and peacefulness, oneness with nature, oneself, and "god." It speaks of things in such an exalted manner that it gives the impression that you have reached a higher plain of thought and understanding. Just as Eve believed when she sinned against God. These feelings are only the cloaks that Satan hides behind. **This is why it is so important to act from principle and not from feelings.** We must live by *"every word that procedeth out of the mouth of God." (Matt. 4:4)* This new philosophy undermines, literally, every principle of Christ. Jesus is not looked upon as your Creator, Saviour, or Friend. It teaches that God is not a personal, loving God, but is an essence found in nature, in you, and in all things. I urge you, not to get entangled in this demon inspired philosophy.

Now it's time for us to look at some of the disciplines in the health care field which we must question.

1. **Acupuncture** - "Acupuncture is thought to be effective by 'unblocking' disturbances within an external energy system. This concept is completely unrelated to the anatomical system of nerves, veins, arteries, and lymphatics that has been carefully documented by scientists of all races and religions and medical centers all over the world." *(Warren Peters, MD. - Mystical Medicine p. 40)* When you ask for concrete anatomic or physiologic data to substantiate these external energy systems; only nebulous, vague, unproven theories are related. Might it work? Of course, but who is the power behind the apparent healing?

2. **Reflexology** - "Reflexology is a close cousin to

acupuncture. Even though seen as a more acceptable 'Western variety' of the energy-balancing technique, its roots are deeply planted in the soil of spiritism. In fact, the same meridian lines of acupuncture apply to reflexology." *(Ibid. page 43)* These meridians have no anatomical or physiological basis. They embrace no true science and are spiritualistic in nature. But which spirit is behind them?

3. **Iridology** - Dr. Carter, a practitioner of iridology states, "Intuitive skills do come into play here, and whether we want to call this 'psychic' ability or not (it remains to be defined)....What do we mean by 'psychic'? Is that just a paranormal state? It is very easy to label it as such. We may find that these skills are just a further progression of the conscious ability of an individual,...a kind of hyperconscious or ulltraconscious state." *(Ibid)* This is not a true science, one which anyone who studies is able to grasp. You must have a "psychic ability"! But who gives you this ability?"

4. **Homeopathy** - Samuel Christian Hahnemann, the father of homeopathy, stated that "like heals like." He stated in his original paper of 1796 that, "The natural disease is never to be considered as noxious material situated somewhere within the interior or exterior of man but as one produced by an inimical spirit-like agency which, like a kind of infection disturbs in its instinctive existence of the spirit-like (conceptual) principle of life within the organism, torturing it as an evil spirit, and compelling it to produce certain ailments and disorders in the regular course of it life"

(Hahnemann, op. cit., p.215). Do you understand that? I don't!☺ Homeopathy states that the more a substance is diluted, the stronger its effect. If you put one teaspoon of sugar in a gallon of water, then take a teaspoon of that mixture and place it in another gallon of water, repeating this process 100 times; then this will result in a final product that is the sweetest of all, right? NOT!☺

5. **Chiropractics** - D. D. Palmer, the founder of chiropractic therapy was highly influenced by Anton Mesmer. He believed that the "life force" communicated through the nerves of the spinal cord. His son B. J. Palmer developed his father's observations into a system of health. He states, "While trying to find my way out of these dilemmas, I took a new look at the basic chiropractic concept of 'innate.' This philosophy insisted that the primal source of energy or vital force (innate) is directed through the nervous system,...innate was that power which keep the complicated autonomic system functioning. Innate was Infinite Life expressing itself through an individual for a specific period of time and space." *(Weldon, Jonh and Wison, Clifford, Occult Shock and Psychic forces. P193-194.)* Our Creator keeps the heart beating and the nervous system functioning. Not innate!

6. **Allopathic Medicine** - Hippocrates, the father of Greek medicine "was of the order of Asclepiade, a guild of physicians believed to be priest of Asklepios, the god of healing. The first oath of the famous Hippocratic oath reads: 'I swear by healing Apollo, by

Asklepios... and by all the gods and goddesses...."" *(Vasquez, M., The Journal of Health & Healing; 19(1), p.16-17)* Allopathic medicine has an occult background. Alchemist, the original physicians, tried to blend base metal into gold, black into white, and good with evil. Pharmakeia, is the Greek word for pharmacy, and means sorcery. Look at any Physician's Desk Reference and you will see that all drugs have side effects. For instance, the diabetes drug Rezulin, manufactured by Parke-Davis is reportedly to have caused 38 cases of acute liver failure with 28 deaths occurring because of its use. It has not been withdrawn from the market. *(New York Times, March 27, 1999)*

In another article in the *New York Times* dated November 30, 1999, the National Academy of Sciences reported that between **44,000 and 98,000 deaths occur each year due to medical mistakes primarily occurring in hospitals.** That exceeds the deaths cause by highway accidents, breast cancer and AIDS combined. So stay out of hospitals whenever possible, if you want to live a longer and healthier life. Allopathic medicine today, uses sound physiologic principles, but because of its strong reliance upon drug medications, it is not the "BEST WAY."

7. **Herbal Medicine** - This is a very enticing discipline because herbs were placed on the earth, by God, for the good of man. I use and prescribe herbs for my patients and know that they are beneficial in the prevention and treatment of disease. But there are herbalist who will try to convince you that their "concoction or formula" is the only one that truly works. There are also

formulas containing a multitude of different herbs, usually very costly, that are "guaranteed" to make you want to feel better." You do eventually feel better, but in many instances, in spite of the preparation you have taken. Certain herbs have side-effects, which may be significant. An article in a medical journal warned about the rapidly progressive kidney failure that was associated with the Chinese herbal remedies, Mu ton and Fanjii. Two patients progressed to end-stage kidney failure. *(Lord, GM; The Lancet 1999;354;481-482,494)* Know also that marijuana and cocaine come from herbs. ☺

Another commonly used herb, Goldenseal, when used for prolonged periods may lead to liver failure.

I encourage the use of simple herbs that are safe, effective, and inexpensive. Follow the guidelines listed to minimize the dangers that some herbs pose.

GUIDELINES FOR THE SAFE USE OF HERBAL TEAS

1. Herbal teas should not be considered cure-alls.

2. Be alert to the toxicity of certain herbs.

3. Beware of unlabeled "loose" or bulk teas.

4. Read labels carefully so that only prepackaged teas with safe ingredients are used.

5. Use only those teas with safe constituents. For minor ailments, use these teas in a therapeutic, and not a prophylactic fashion.

6. Do not take more than four herbs at any one time.

7. Drink no more than 1-2 cups of herbal tea per day on a regular basis. The long term effects of drinking most herbal teas in large quantities are not known.

8. People who have an allergic response to ragweed, asters, or chrysanthemums should avoid all teas containing marigold, yarrow, and chamomile flowers.

9. Pregnant women should especially use caution in drinking any herbal teas since few have been thoroughly tested for safety. A pregnant woman should consult with her physician prior to using herbal teas. Likewise, young children should restrict their use of herbal teas.

10. USE HERBAL TEAS ONLY FOR SPECIFIC MEDICAL PURPOSES. THEY MUST NOT BE USED AS A SUBSTITUTE FOR A COMPETENT MEDICAL EVALUATION.

(Craig, WJ, The Use and Safety of Common Herbs and Herbal Teas, Golden Harvest Books, Second Edition, 1996, p.37)

8. **Hypnosis** - Of all the possible counterfeits to true healing, hypnosis is one of the most insidious and dangerous. Scripture says, *"Let this mind be in you, which was also in Christ Jesus"; (Philippians 2:5).* Hypnosis places your mind under the control of a fallible, sinful human being. Even if the motives are honorable, this is a very dangerous proposition. To surrender your mind to the unconscious insinuations and suggestions of any human being is not wise. Being fully conscious of what is going into your mind at all times is imperative. You should yield your mind only to Jesus Christ!

I remember an experience I had, during my residency training, when a clinical psychologist used hypnosis to "help" a Christian lady come out of her "restrictive shell." This lady began going to night clubs, then she started drinking alcoholic beverages. Soon, she became very promiscuous. He thought he had done her a great service when, in fact, he caused her to become the slave of Satan.

Some use hypnosis for things like helping others to stop smoking. This sounds, on the surface, like a worthy purpose. But this causes the smoker to look to a man, rather than to God for success. Another one of Satan's tricks. Do not, I repeat, do not surrender your will to anyone but Jesus!

I would like to interject right here, that many honest, sincere, and caring people believe in and are practicing these forms of healing. But sincerity is not the test for truth. They are sincerely wrong. This is why the Holy Spirit tells us through the apostle John what is truth. *"Sanctify them through thy truth: thy word is truth."(John 17:17)*

"There are many ways of practicing the healing art, but there is only one way that Heaven approves. God's remedies are the simple agencies of nature that will not tax or debilitate the system through their powerful properties. Pure air and water, cleanliness, a proper diet, purity of life and a firm trust in God, are remedies for the want of which thousands are dying, yet these remedies are going out of date because their skillful use requires work that the people do not appreciate." *(E. G. White, Testimonies to the Church, volume 5, p.443)*

God's remedies will lead you to a greater love, a closer relationship, and a greater appreciation for your Creator, Jesus Christ; and not to a mystical belief in a spirit or an essence.

Remember, *"There is a way that seemeth right unto a man, but the end thereof are the ways of death."(Proverbs 16:25)* Satan in these last days is seeking to deceive and destroy. You will hear things that sound good, that *"seemeth right."* It may even help you; but remember the text ends with this warning; *"but the end thereof are the ways of death."* God's Word, I say again, must be the yardstick by which you measure all things. May God grant you His Holy Spirit, that you may not be deceived by the spirits of devils!

CHAPTER 7

COMMON DISEASES AND THEIR TREATMENT

"And great multitudes came unto him, having with them those that were lame, blind, dumb, maimed, and many others, and cast them down at Jesus' feet; and he healed them:" Matthew 15:30

The **BEST WAY** program will help in the prevention and treatment of most, if not all of the diseases and illnesses we face. We will now consider several common health problems and give very practical suggestions on how to treat them. Some of these conditions require professional expertise to manage, and I strongly advise you to consult your primary care physician for their management.

111

HYPERTENSION

Hypertension causes few symptoms, thus it is called "the silent killer." Most people feel perfectly fine during the early stages of this disease. Yet, if left undetected and untreated, hypertension can contribute to diseases of the heart and blood vessels, especially those in the brain. Blindness and kidney failure are also associated with hypertension. **YOU MUST GET YOUR BLOOD PRESSURE CHECKED REGULARLY!** Poor diet, lack of exercise, obesity, anxiety, quarreling, and other emotional distress can cause blood pressure elevation. Blood pressure, thus elevated, may remain high even if it fluctuates up and down for a time.

In the United States, hypertension is directly or indirectly related to more diseases and disabilities than any other medical condition. Between 10-30% of Americans have elevated blood pressure. Over 30% of Black Americans have hypertension. In those over 64 years old, one out of every two has hypertension. It is the #1 cause of death among Blacks in America.

But just what is hypertension? Hypertension is defined as a sustained blood pressure of 140/90 or above. The top number is called the systolic blood pressure and is the maximal pressure exerted by the heart (the left ventricle to be specific), when it contracts. The bottom number or diastolic blood pressure, is the pressure on the heart while it is resting between beats.

HYPERTENSION MUST BE CONTROLLED! Seek medical attention if your blood pressure remains higher than 140/90 on three separate occasions, on three separate days, outside of the doctor's office.

Do you want to control your blood pressure? The BEST WAY may be the only intervention you need. It's worth a try! Let's see how the program works.

♦ **Bedtime regularity** - this helps you to handle stress more appropriately. While sleeping the blood pressure decreases, reducing the stress on the heart. 7-8 hours of sleep are best.

♦ **Exercise** is important in keeping the blood vessels in a healthy tone. Walking at a moderate pace, and useful labor, such as gardening, for about 20-30 minutes, will reduce blood pressure. Exercise 4-6 times each week.

♦ **Sunshine** helps the body metabolize calcium better and is known to be beneficial in decreasing blood pressure.

♦ **Simple diet** is essential. Some believe that a high intake of potassium from fruits and vegetables is important. I recommend that my patients with hypertension eat 5 servings of fruit, and 3-5 servings of vegetables each day.

Sodium, is one of the elements in salt and must be greatly reduced. Foods that contain more than 150 mg. of sodium per serving should not be used regularly. Read the labels on all processed and canned foods because they are usually very high in sodium.

Cheese is very detrimental because of its high sodium and fat content. I recommend that you dispense with its use. (See recipes for a tasty and healthful cheese substitute.)

♦ **Temperance** is vital. When you are still growing after the age of 20 years old, wider but not taller,☺ you are at risk for developing hypertension. It is believed that for every pound of weight you lose, your blood pressure drops 1 mm. (The principles outlined in the Prudent Diet are ideal for weight reduction. Also see "Winning the Battle of the Bulge" later in this chapter.)

Alcohol is definitely bad news, especially when it comes to   hypertension. No one with or without hypertension should use alcoholic beverages of any kind. *Caffeine* and *tobacco* also elevate blood pressure, so stay away from both of them.

♦ **Water** is essential in keeping the blood from becoming too thick. Drink at least 6-8 glasses/day unless you are on fluid restriction. Do not be concerned that drinking water will cause fluid retention. The reason we retain fluid is not because of the water we drink, but because we are using too much sodium. And where sodium goes so does water. Diuretics or fluid pills remove sodium from the body through the kidneys and affect water indirectly. So enjoy Adam's Ale.☺

Hydrotherapy is beneficial in improving blood vessel tone and is therefore helpful in the treatment of hypertension. The treatment I recommend most for my patients whose blood pressure is not above, 160/95 is the contrast shower. (See the section on hydrotherapy.)

♦ **Air** - Deep, slow breathing has been shown to be very calming and is a technique that should be used in any stressful situation. This helps to decrease the blood pressure elevation associated with stress, tension, and anxiety.

♦ **Yielding Trust in God's Power.** To accomplish any of the above you need Jesus. Ask Him for the help that only He can give. Then yield to His all-knowing wisdom and trust His matchless love. He will give you success. *"Delight thyself also in the LORD; and he shall give thee the desires of thine heart." (Ps 37:4)*

Clinical Case #1: A 49-year-old Black male with a long history of "borderline" hypertension, was placed on antihypertensive medication one week prior to coming into my office for a consultation. He did not want to take the medication. His initial blood pressure was 156/100. He started the BEST WAY program, and was seen for a follow-up visit one month later. His blood pressure at that time was 140/90 on no medications. He had lost 14 pounds and was "feeling great." His blood pressures at home were running between 116/70 and 130/83. The patient continues to do well at the time of the writing of this book. GOD IS ABLE!

Clinical Case #2: A 48-year-old Black male had a 15-month history of hypertension. Three different medications were used in an attempt to control the blood pressure, but side-effects made their use unacceptable. One medication had even caused an elevation in his liver enzymes. Home blood pressures on the medications stayed around 130/86. When off the medications his blood pressure was around 150/95. He came to my office for a consultation desiring a non pharmacologic approach to this problem. His initial blood pressure was 148/98. His weight was 242½ pounds. The patient also complained of easy irritability, arthritis pain in his fingers, and increased stress. He was placed on the

BEST WAY program and seen in follow-up one month later. At that time his blood pressure was 142/86 on no medication. His primary care physician, whom he had seen two weeks earlier, had discontinued the medication because of the improvement in his blood pressure. He also lost 15 pounds. The arthritis pain in his fingers had completely stopped. His wife noticed a significant improvement in his ability of handling job and church stress. (The patient is a minister). He related that even his parishioners had noticed a greater spirituality in his sermons. The patient has continued to do well. TO GOD BE THE GLORY!

DIABETES MELLITUS

Commonly called "sugar," diabetes mellitus afflicts between 7-10 million Americans. It is estimated that another 7-10 million Americans have diabetes but are not aware of it. This means that one in every 17 adults or 6% of the population in this country has diabetes. There are another 35-40 million adults that have what is termed, impaired glucose tolerance. They have an increased risk of developing diabetes. So you can see this is not a small problem.

Certain ethnic groups have a greater risk for this illness. Pima Indians, Hispanics, Blacks, and Asians have a rate that is 1 ½ to two times greater than whites.

Diabetes causes a substantial increase in morbidity and mortality. This is due to the coronary artery disease and kidney failure that is associated with the disease. Diabetes is the leading cause of blindness, kidney failure, and lower extremity amputations in the United States. The pain of diabetic neuropathy is disheartening to many. Mortality rates in diabetics are two to four times higher than those of non diabetics.

But just what is diabetes? Diabetes mellitus is a disease which affects glucose metabolism. It is diagnosed when the blood glucose or sugar is 126 mg/dl. or above, following an eight to 12-hour fast. This test should be repeated on three occasions prior to making a definitive diagnosis of diabetes mellitus. Normal fasting blood sugar values range between 70-110 mg/dl. Impaired glucose tolerance is defined as a fasting blood glucose of between 111-125 mg/dl. If your blood sugar is above normal, you are at risk of developing a plethora of physical problems.

117

There are two types of diabetes; Type 1 and 2. Type 1 was previously called juvenile-onset diabetes or insulin dependent diabetes because it usually occurs prior to the age of 20 years. It is due to inadequate amounts of insulin being produced by the pancreas. Type 1 is believed to be caused by a viral infection occurring early in life. The virus destroys the beta cells of the Islets or Langerhann which are responsible for the production of insulin. Another theory is that Type 1 diabetes is an autoimmune disease, meaning that the body's own immune system destroys these cells. Cows' milk has been implicated by some to be responsible for this immune problem, because the protein in cows' milk is similar to that found in human milk. *(Scott FW. Cow milk and insulin-dependent diabetes mellitus: is there a relationship? American Journal of Clinical Nutrition, 1990;51:489-91.) (Karjalainen J, Martin JM, Kmip M, et al. A bovine Albumin peptide as a possible tripper of insulin-dependent diabetes mellitus. New England Journal of Medicine 1992:327:302-7.)* This type of diabetes comprises approximately 10% of all known diabetics.

Type 2 diabetes, also called adult-onset or non-insulin dependent diabetes, is not due to an inadequate amount of insulin, but to the insulin not working properly. There is usually a strong family history associated with this condition. It was called adult-onset because it usually started after the age of 40 years old. It was called non-insulin dependent because a person is able to do very well without the use of insulin. Type 2 diabetes accounts for approximately 90% of known diabetics.

But just how does insulin work? We can liken insulin to the keys which unlock doors, allowing glucose to move from the blood stream into the cells for metabolism. This reduces the

blood glucose. In Type 1 diabetes there are not enough keys to open enough doors to move the glucose out of the blood stream into the cells. Therefore, the blood sugars stay above 125 mg/dl. In Type 2 diabetes, there are plenty of keys, but the locks are defective. Consequently, the glucose remains in the blood stream driving the fasting sugar above 125 mg/dl.
Signs and symptoms of diabetes include constant thirst and urination, weight loss even though there has not been a change in diet, fatigue, recurrent yeast infections, slow wound healing, and decreased vision. If you have a family member with diabetes and/or have any of these symptoms you should be evaluated by your primary care physician as soon as possible.

Type 2 diabetes is primarily caused by unhealthy lifestyle practices. These include, inappropriate dietary habits, such as eating too much fat, and not getting adequate amounts of exercise; which leads to obesity. Making simple lifestyle changes will lead to either a cure, a reversal, or a significant improvement in this disease. Type 2 diabetes is even on the rise among teens and children, due to the sedentary lifestyle and dietary habits that our society has adopted. If you are overweight at the age of 25, you have a three fold greater risk of developing diabetes in your 50's, than if you are normal weight at age 25. *(Archives of Internal Medicine 1999;159:957-963)*.

WARNING: Before you embark on any program, you should consult your primary care physician.

All medications including those used to treat diabetes have side-effects. One medication, Rezulin, has been linked to 38 deaths. It is therefore best to take a lifestyle approach first in the preventions and treatment of this disease.

The lifestyle program that I recommend is, you guessed it, the ***BEST WAY!***☺

♦ **Bedtime regularity** allows you to get the rest needed to handle stress more effectively. Stress increases blood glucose levels even under ideal circumstances. Getting to bed early also helps to prevent late night eating, which is definitely detrimental.

♦ **Exercise** is a very important factor in treating and reversing this disease. Studies show that exercise repairs the insulin receptors, the locks, allowing the keys, insulin, to unlock and open the doors. This reduces the blood sugar level. In a large multi center trial, participants who were physically active, had better insulin activity, than their sedentary counterparts. This improved the utilization of glucose by muscle cells resulting in lower blood glucose levels. *(Medical Tribune: Internist & Cardiologist Editions 39(8); 1998).* Another study revealed that walking was as beneficial as more vigorous exercise in diabetics, if the duration was the same. *(Journal of the American Medical Association 1998:279:669-674).* With proper exercise, you just may be able to "walk away" from your diabetes. ☺

Gestational diabetics, those who develop the disease while they are pregnant, may be able to avoid insulin injections and medications, if they exercise. This may even prevent the occurrence of Type 2 diabetes later in life which happens commonly in gestational diabetics. Those women who were active prior to becoming pregnant, were less likely to develop diabetes during their pregnancy. *(Family Practice News; September 15, 1999)* **SO GET UP AND GET MOVING, FOR YOUR HEALTH!**

♦ **Sunshine** - One of the known benefits of sunshine is improved muscular performance. This improves the muscles utilization of glucose, and helps reduce the blood glucose levels

♦ **Simple Diet** - Many Type 2 diabetics have this disease because they are overweight and consume too many calories. Diabetes is associated with a high dietary fat intake, more than with any other type of food. We recommend a high complex carbohydrate vegan diet, with very little added fat. Free fats, in the form of oils, margarine, spreads, etc. must be avoided. No fried foods should be consumed if you are diabetic. Eat only two (2) meals each day, if it is approved by your primary care physician. **Do not make this dietary change until you see your physician.**

♦ **Temperance** - Because 90% of Type 2 diabetics are overweight, it is imperative to eat moderately. You must totally abstain from alcohol, caffeine and tobacco. All are harmful for diabetics.

♦ **Water** is very important in preventing dehydration. It contains no calories and is of great benefit in the prevention and treatment of diabetes. I recommend, as stated earlier, that you drink 6-8 glasses each day (8 oz glasses). But be careful. If you are always thirty, it could be that your blood sugars are not being adequately controlled.

♦ **Air** - All diabetics must breathe, this will prolong your life.☺ Deep breathing, of fresh air, as fresh as your environment provides, improves circulation. This is important in diabetics because of their predilection for peripheral vascular diseases (circulatory problems in their extremities).

♦ **Yielding Trust in God's Power** - Because Type 2 diabetes is a lifestyle disease, it must be managed with lifestyle interventions. I'm reminded of the text, *"Can the Ethiopian change his skin, or the leopard his spots? then may ye also do good, that are accustomed to do evil."* *(Jeremiah 13:23)* From this text, you may readily discern that you need God's divine power to makes positive changes. So don't be discouraged because of former failures. Trust in Jesus, and He will surely do for you those things which you are unable to do for yourself. *"For I can do all things through Christ that strengheneth me."(Philippians 4:13)* **TRUST IN THE LORD YOUR GOD AND HE WILL BRING IT TO PAST!**

Clinical Case: A 51-year-old Black female with a 20 year history of Type 2 diabetes came to the office for a consultation. She weighed 290 lbs. and was taking 70 units of insulin every day. She was also taking 14 other medications for one or several of the following problems: hypertension, elevated cholesterol, asthma, joint swelling, swelling of her ankles, an enlarged heart, hypothyroidism (an underactive thyroid gland), gastroesophageal reflux disease, and diabetic neuropathy, (a condition characterized by numbness, tingling, and pain in the lower and upper extremities.) She had attended our community health seminars. She diligently followed the BEST WAY program and 10 months later, her weight was 210 lbs., and her fasting blood sugars were between 74-100 mg/dl on only 5 units of insulin per day. Her blood pressure was better controlled on 1/4 the dosage of medications. She has no problems with acid reflux, asthma or ankle edema now. Her neuropathy and cholesterol levels have improved. We praise and thank God for her faithfulness and His blessings. Remember, with God, "ALL THINGS ARE POSSIBLE."

CANCER

"Is there anything too hard for the Lord?" (Genesis 18:14)

Cancer is a group of diseases characterized by the uncontrolled growth of abnormal cells. It may occur in any tissue or organ of the body.

The risk factors for cancer include:
1. A genetic predisposition.
2. An immune system compromise.
3. Certain lifestyle habits.

While we cannot do anything, at this point, about the genetic predisposition to cancer; we are able to improve the function of our immune system and correct those lifestyle habits that put us at risk for cancer. Let's consider the benefits of the BEST WAY, in cancer prevention and treatment.

♦ **Bedtime regularity** - For the immune system to function properly you must get adequate sleep. 7-8 hours are optimal.

♦ **Exercise** - The beneficial effect of exercise on white blood cell function is universally accepted. Exercise is known to enhance the production of endorphins, which are hormones that improve the functions of natural killer T-lymphocytes. Intemperance with exercise, too much and too often, may actually suppress immune system functions. Walking for 20-30 minutes each day would be ideal and not considered intemperate.☺

♦ **Sunshine** - As we have already discussed, proper exposure to sunlight is beneficial for the psyche and for the body's

124

immune system through vitamin D metabolism.

♦ **Simple diet** - For any cancer prevention or treatment program, a VEGETARIAN DIET is best. God's original diet for man, was vegetarian (See Genesis 1:29). 80% of bowel, breast, and prostate cancers are related to diet. "Cancers, tumors, and all inflammatory diseases are largely caused by meat eating. From the light God has given me, the prevalence of cancer and tumors is largely due to gross living on dead flesh." *(White, E.G., Counsel on Diets and Foods: p.388)*

Dairy products should also be eliminated. Soy products are far superior in every way. Cow's milk is best for baby cows. ☺

The diet must include 3-5 servings of vegetables every day. Broccoli, kale, brussels sprouts, and cauliflower have been shown to protect the body against certain types of cancer. *(American Journal of Clinical Nutrition: 1999;69:712-718)* Tomatoes are stated to be beneficial in preventing prostate cancer. It is my belief that they will also help to prevent other forms of cancer.

You should eat largely of whole grains, including whole wheat, barley, rye, oats, brown rice and corn. Whole grains should be eaten every day to the tune of 6-11 servings.

Fruits are also important, the more, the better. I recommend you eat 5 servings of fruit each day because of their therapeutic phytochemicals.

Legumes or beans help to eliminate carcinogens from the body because of their high fiber content. Eat dry beans 5-7 times each week.

Fried foods, butter, and margarine, should be avoided. Many forms of cancer are associated with a high fat intake. They include breast, colon, and prostate cancers. Animal fats especially pose a risk. *(Journal of the National Cancer Institute 1999:91:414-428)*

Eliminate high sugar foods like soft drinks and candies. I do not recommend artificial sweeteners because they may adversely affect your immune system. Restrict sweets to natural, unrefined products. Eliminate white sugar. Sucanat is an excellent sweetener and is also very nutritious.

♦ **Temperance** - Alcohol, tobacco, and caffeine are all risk factors for cancer in one form or another. Obesity and stress are associated with cancer cell initiation and immune system compromise.

♦ **Water** - Hydrotherapy is used as an immune stimulant. I recommend some form of hydrotherapy for all of my cancer patients. The hot tub baths, short cold baths, or contrast showers are the treatments of choice. To do a short cold bath or shower, start with the temperature around 90 degrees for 5-15 minutes and gradually decrease the temperature over several weeks to 75 degrees for 5-15 minutes. If you have angina pectoris, avoid this treatment!

♦ **Air** - Deep breathing acts as a stress reducer. We

recommend three deep breaths, three times each day.

♦ **Yielding Trust in God's Power** - Faith has a beneficial effect on our entire body as we have already discovered. Remember the promise, *"Bless the Lord, O my soul; and all that is within me, bless His holy name. Bless the Lord, O my soul and forget not all of His benefits: Who forgiveth all thine iniquities; who healeth all thy diseases. (Psalms 103:1-3)*

Other helpful modalities include:
♦ Herbal therapies: Red Clover, Flaxseed, Garlic, Turmeric, Ginger, Sage, Thyme, Oregano, Basil, Licorice and Gotu Kola are excellent immune stimulants and contain phytochemicals with anti cancer properties *(Craig, WJ, The Use and Safety of Common Herbs and Herbal Teas, Golden Harvest Books, Second Edition, 1996, p.37)*. One cup of tea each day made from any of the above herbs is helpful. You should use them as seasonings whenever possible. Simple herbs may be a part of any cancer prevention or treatment program. If you have cancer, then larger amounts may be used. Consult with your physician for assistance.

♦ Activated charcoal may also help. Making slurry water for drinking or enemas will adsorb excessive gas and toxins. It will do no harm, only good. You make slurry water by mixing one teaspoon of activated charcoal with eight oz. of water. Allow the charcoal to settle and drink the water off the top. You may also use charcoal capsules or tablets. It is used in emergency rooms to adsorb drugs and medications when an overdose occurs.

WARNING: ACTIVATED CHARCOAL IS NOT THE SAME AS THE BRIQUETS USED IN GRILLING!

ClinicalCase #1: A 54-year-old Black male with lung cancer had undergone surgery for the removal of the primary mass. He was started on chemotherapy but was unable to complete the full regimen due to the bone marrow suppression caused by the chemotherapy. He attended one of our community seminars with his wife, and they came to the office for a consultation. He was placed on the BEST WAY program, and was subsequently able to complete the full chemotherapy course without any suppression of his white blood cell count. The patient is doing fine as of the writing of this book.

Clinical Case #2: A 32-year-old Black female noticed soreness in her right leg and was diagnosed with a blood clot (thrombophlebitis). She was later found to have a soft tissue malignancy in her right leg, a leiomyosarcoma, with liver involvement. Chemotherapy was recommended but she declined this option, and presented to my office one month post diagnosis, for a consultation. She was placed on the BEST WAY program and was seen one month later for follow-up. At that time she was doing well. Her oncologist from Johns Hopkins University was sympathetic with her desire to forgo chemotherapy. Her oncologist saw her two months later and wanted to know what she was doing. The MRI of her liver showed definite regression of the tumor. She shared with her the BEST WAY program which was accepted by the oncologist without hesitancy. As of the writing of this book she is doing well. TO GOD BE THE GLORY!

WINNING THE BATTLE OF THE BULGE!

"And take heed to yourselves, lest at any time your hearts be overcharged with surfeiting , and drunkenness, and the cares of this life, and so that day come upon you unawares." (Luke 21:34)

In this land of plenty, the United States, we are truly showing our prosperity in inappropriate ways. The most common manifestation of this prosperity is obesity. 34 million Americans are obese. And 11 million are markedly obese. The poor and minorities have the highest rate of obesity. Obesity is on the rise among children and teenagers. Obesity is associated with higher rates of practically every chronic disease. Hypertension, diabetes mellitus, gallstones, heart disease, osteoarthritis, surgical complications, and certain forms of cancers all share obesity as a common denominator. To reduce the probability of suffering from one or more of these diseases, reducing your weight by correcting your lifestyle is the most prudent strategy.

Just what is obesity? Obesity is defined as being 20% above your ideal body weight (IBW), or having a body mass index (BMI) of 29 or greater for females, and 30 or greater for males. But what is my IBW? In the book *"Nutrition of Vegetarians,"* Drs. Thrash offers a simple formula for calculating your IBW. For females, allow 100 lbs. for the first five feet of height, and add 5 pounds for each additional inch. For males allow 100 lbs. for the first 5 feet of height, and 7 lbs. for each additional inch. Example: A 6 foot male should weight 184 lbs. (100 lbs. for the first 5 feet, and 7 lbs. for each additional inch. 100+84=184 lbs.) 20% of this, would add an additional 36 lbs. Therefore if he weighed over 220 lbs., he would be obese.

While this is not an exact science, it provides a general idea of what your weight should be.

But I must inform you, that the excessive **weight is not, never has been, and never will be the problem. It's only a symptom of the problem!** Any attempt to control the symptom only, by going on a special diet, taking pills or herbal formulas, or using other highly questionable techniques such as acupuncture, acupressure, etc.; is doomed for long term failure. You can lose weight following almost any special diet, high protein or not, but it will only be "for a season." I know individuals that have lost over 300 pounds in their lifetime and they weigh over 300 pounds now. This occurs because short-term modifications, which are not accompanied by changes in the lifestyle, will be just that, short termed. You must address the problem, **the unhealthy lifestyle**.

Because of time and space constraints, I will briefly address the impact of the BEST WAY program on weight management. If you follow these principles, long-term success over this health destroying condition is assured.

♦ **Bedtime regularity** is vital if you want to lose weight. If you stay up too late, after 10:00 p.m., you will be tempted to eat late. And one of the major causes of obesity is late night eating. So go to bed, not to dinner during the night!☺

♦ **Exercise** - Inactivity is also a major contributor to obesity. In years gone by, we were more active. We walked more and drove less; we climbed stairs instead of riding elevators and escalators; we participated in more physical activities and watched television less; and we pushed the lawnmower instead of riding it. Therefore, we were more "slim and trim" instead of being "flabby and shabby."☺ Walking to the store, taking the stairs instead of the elevator, raking the leaves instead of blowing them, vacuuming the carpet more often, are all forms of exercise which keeps the metabolic rate from declining when calories are restricted. It is not necessary to join a health club, nor is it necessary to get the heart rate up to 70% of the predicted maximal rate for your age for 20-30 minutes. Walking for a total of 30 minutes each day is best, even if it's done in 10 minute intervals. In fact, any activity that burns calories is helpful.

♦ **Sunshine:** We encourage you to get sun exposure daily, because of its beneficial effects. The sun warms the body, increasing its metabolic rate. Even though this is not a significant factor in weight loss, it can only help. Sunshine also helps you to ward off feelings of depression.

♦ **Simple Diet** is the cornerstone of any successful weight management program. God placed in food, a natural barrier to overeating. That barrier is **FIBER,** the non-digestible part of plants. We lose this very beneficial substance when plant foods are refined. There is no fiber in animal products, and many people lose weight simply by eating more fruits, legumes, whole grains, and vegetables.

The other factors I want to mention are fats, between meal snacks, not eating a good breakfast, and eating heavy suppers. These factors will definitely sabotage your quest to become "less of yourself."☺

Fats contain two and one-half times the calories of carbohydrates and proteins. Because of this, it is a potent effector of obesity. To avoid fats, you must read food labels. If the fat calories constitute more than 25% or 1/4 of the total calories, then that item should be left on the shelf, in the majority of cases. Cookies, baked goods, along with ready to eat foods are usually very high in fat. Frying is a fast and easy way to get unwanted calories. Frying pans may be used for anything, with one exception, frying!☺ (See the section on fat in the Prudent Diet for other information.)

Between Meal Snacks: "How many of you eat healthy snacks?" is a question I ask during many of the seminars I conduct or participate in. Hands usually go flying up all over the room. This gives me the opportunity of informing the participants that, "there is no such thing as a healthy snack!"☺ (Except in very rare circumstances.) In the media this obesity inducing habit is advanced by the "snack food" industry for monetary reasons alone and not for your health.

In addition to its impact on obesity, this habit is a major contributor to the epidemic of digestive related problems in our society. These include: indigestion, esophageal reflux disease, heartburn, constipation, bloating, diarrhea, and the like. Even foods that are considered "healthy snacks," which is a misnomer because no snacks are healthy, will cause you to be more of yourself than you desire. In fact, just drinking one glass of juice each day, approximately 100 calories, if not used for energy or burned up, will cause as much as a 10 lb. weight gain in one year. And who drinks only one glass of juice?

The only safe between meal "snack" is water! I advise you to drink 6-8 glasses of water each day, unless you are on fluid restrictions. "But I don't like water!" you may say. "What does that have to do with anything?"☺ You should not drink water because you like it, but because its best for your body. You must act from principle and not because of your likes and dislikes.

WARNING: If you have diabetes, and are on medications, it may be dangerous to eliminate between meal snacks! Please consult with your physician first!

Breakfast and Supper: To be successful in managing your weight, you must eat a substantial and nutritious breakfast **every** day. This allows you to metabolize the calories consumed more efficient, before the body converts them to fat. Calories are needed when you are going to be most active, not when you are going to sleep. If a third meal is eaten, it should be very light. Though it would be best to eat only two (2) meals a day. When God fed men, they ate two meals per day; (see 1 Kings 17:6, Exodus 16:12.)

♦ **Temperance** - Do not overeat! When you have had enough, don't try to see how much you can eat before it affects your breathing. I remember attending a dinner, where a friend was asked, "Have you had enough?" He jokingly replied after taking a deep breath, "No I haven't, I can still breathe."☺ Eat only as much food as is necessary for you to get to the next meal without becoming famished. Remember, one of the Fruits of the Spirit is **TEMPERANCE!**

♦   **Water** - is the drink that contains no calories and will reduce the sensations of hunger. You should drink 6-8 glasses each day, between meals.

♦   **Air** - Deep breathing is a stress reducer. It is especially helpful for those who use food to cope with stress.

♦   **Yielding Trust in God** - God can and will give you success. It is impossible to eat right without God's help, so pray that you will be strengthened to follow these simple guidelines. *"I can do all things through Christ which strengheneth me."(Philippians 4:13)*

Clinical Case #1: A 51 year old Black female who during a ten month period of following the BEST WAY program, lost over 80 pounds (from 290 lbs. to 210 lbs.) As of the writing of this book she is doing very well.

Clinical Case #2: A 64-year-old Black female who after 9 months on the BEST WAY program, lost 28 pounds (from 169 lbs. to 141 lbs.) She continues to do well and her weight is stable at the time this book was written.

HEART DISEASE

"And I will give them one heart, and I will put a new spirit within you; and I will take away the stony heart out of their flesh, and will give them an heart of flesh." (Ezekiel 11:19)

Heart disease is the #1 killer of Americans. Each year 33% of all deaths in the U.S. occur because of coronary artery disease. Annually 954,000 Americans die secondary to diseases of the heart and blood vessels. Over 1.5 million myocardial infarctions (heart attacks) occur each year. *(Benitex, RM, Atherosclerosis; An Infectious Disease?, Hospital Practice; 9/1/1999).* The sad fact is, the majority of these cases occur because we disregard basic health principles. Risk factors for heart disease are hypertension, diabetes, high cholesterol, and others.

CHOLESTEROL

Cholesterol, a white, waxy, fat-like substance is found all over the body and is essential to life. Cholesterol is partly responsible for you and me being here today, because it is the substrate from which the body produces its sex hormones. So we NEED cholesterol!☺ But how much must we have in our diets to be healthy? ABSOLUTELY NONE! The body produces all the cholesterol we need, in the liver. And of course this is the case! If it were not, then cholesterol containing foods would have been a part of the original diet.

An elevated blood cholesterol is one of the major risk factors in the development of coronary artery disease. Cholesterol is only found in animal products. Among populations where animal products are not eaten, the incidence of heart disease is dramatically lower. Seventh-day Adventist men in California who were vegan vegetarians, those who ate no animal products at all, had an 86% lower death rate from heart disease than men in the general population. Lacto-ovo vegetarian Adventist men, those that ate no meat but did consume dairy products and eggs, had a mortality rate that was 56% lower men in the general population. *(Scharffenberg, JA, Journal of Health and Healing, Lifestyle Advantage: 1985.)* This demonstrates the impact of dietary cholesterol on heart disease.

There are several types of cholesterol. We will only consider the two main types in this discussion. HDL or high density lipoprotein cholesterol, is the "helpful" or good type. HDL is produced by the liver and actually removes cholesterol deposits from arteries preventing them from becoming blocked or occluded. LDL or low density lipoprotein cholesterol is the "lousy" or bad type and is deposited into the arteries, causing occlusion. So why not just eat the good type of cholesterol? This you cannot do, because no dietary cholesterol is good for you. *(The Wellness Encyclopedia, University of California, Berkeley, 1991; p.41)* And in the majority of cases, there is a direct correlation between the dietary and blood cholesterol levels. Therefore, it is best to eliminate cholesterol from your diet.

The following table list the levels of cholesterol that would increase or reduce your risk for heart disease.

CHOLESTEROL AND HEART DISEASE RISK

Risk of Heart Disease	Total Chol.	LDL Chol.	HDL Chol. Male / Female	HDL/Total Chol. Male / Female
Very Low	100 + age	under 100	>65 / >75	<3.4 / 3.3
Low	under 200	100- 130	55 / 65	4.0 / 3.8
Average	200-225	131-140	45 / 55	5.0 / 4.5
Moderate 2 x average	226-239	141-159	25 / 40	9.5 / 7.0
High 3 x average	>240	>160	<25 / <40	>23 / >11

Adapted from The Wellness Encyclopedia 1991, University of California, Berkeley. P. 43

If your cholesterol levels are in the very low to low risk range, then you are less likely to have a problem with atherosclerosis, though other factors have to be considered (See below).

FACTORS THAT REDUCE CHOLESTEROL!

♦ SOLUBLE FIBER: Lowers cholesterol. Found in beans, oats, fruits, and vegetables,

♦ POLYUNSATURATED FATS: Lowers LDL, "lousy" cholesterol. Found in safflower, sesame, and soybean oils. But use them sparingly.

♦ MONO-UNSATURATED FATS: Lowers cholesterol. Found in olive oil. Use them in moderation.

♦ OMEGA-3 FATTY ACIDS: Lowers total & LDL, "lousy," cholesterol. They are found in flaxseed and cold water fish, although fish are not the best source. This is because fish contains cholesterol. Fish also have a high incidence of cancer in them. *(Scharffenberg, JA, The Whole Story's Fishy, Journal of Health & Healing; Vol.11: No.2; p.16)* Flaxseed, by contrast, is an excellent and inexpensive source of this beneficial fatty acid.

♦ AEROBIC EXERCISE: Regular exercise increases HDL, "helpful" cholesterol.

♦ MAINTAIN PROPER WEIGHT: For every two pounds of excessive weight your total cholesterol is raised by one point (mg/dl.)

♦ AVOID SATURATED FATS: Beef, butter, whole-milk dairy products, dark poultry, poultry skin, and pork, all increase blood cholesterol.

♦ AVOID ANIMAL PRODUCTS: They contain cholesterol.

♦ AVOID TOBACCO USE: Tobacco increases LDL "lousy" cholesterol and decreases HDL "helpful" cholesterol.

(The Wellness Encyclopedia, University of California, Berkeley, 1991; p.41)

HOMOCYSTEINE

Homocysteine is an amino acid used by the body to make proteins and is found in the diet. High levels are associated with an increase in the risk of heart disease. An inadequate intake of the vitamins, folate, B-6, or B-12 may increase homocysteine blood levels. The U.S. Public Health Service recommends 400 mcg. (micrograms) of folate as being optimal in keeping homocysteine levels normal. Good sources of folate are: (½ cup servings, unless otherwise specified)

1.	Product 19 cereal (1 cup)	400 mcg.
2.	Total cereal (3/4 cup)	400
3.	Brewer's yeast (1 T)	313
4.	Lentils (½ cup)	179
5.	Pinto beans or chickpeas	145
6.	Spinach	131
7.	Red kidney beans	115
8.	Asparagus (5 spears)	110

9.	Orange juice (1 cup)	109
10.	Most breakfast cereals	100
11.	Wheat germ (1/4 cup)	100
12.	Split peas	64
13.	Beets	45

(Donna Liebman, Folic Acid: For the Young and Heart, Nutrition Action Health Letter; Vol.27, No.7; Sept. 1995)

You can easily get the recommended amounts of this very important vitamin with the proper dietary approach, reducing the blood levels of homocysteine which decreases the risk of heart disease.

STRESS

Another factor which I must mentioned is the impact of stress on blood cholesterol levels and heart disease. Excessive stress, emotional or physical, causes an elevation in the total and LDL, "lousy," blood cholesterol levels.

Regular, moderate exercise is profitable in handling stress. Every detrimental physiologic change caused by stress, is neutralized by exercise. To cope with the emotional aspect of stress, Jesus has promised, *"Peace I leave with you, my peace I give unto you: not as the world giveth, give I unto you. Let not your heart be troubled, neither let it be afraid." (John 14:27)*

Now let's see how the BEST WAY helps to prevent and treat heart disease.

♦ **Bedtime regularity** - Getting adequate sleep, 7-8 hours each night is optimal. This helps to handle stress more effectively. It also helps to lower the blood pressure which is another risk factor for heart disease.

♦ **Exercise** - The beneficial effect of exercise in raising the HDL, "helpful," cholesterol, has been addressed. Exercise also reduces blood pressure which is another risk factor in heart disease. 20-30 minutes of walking, 4-5 times per week is adequate. Useful labor is one of the best exercises. Stress cannot be handled appropriately without exercise.

♦ **Sunshine** is helpful because it converts cholesterol into a precursor of vitamin D. This reduces the blood cholesterol levels. This effect is quite small, but "every little bit helps."

♦ **Simple diet** - Diet is one of the mainstays in reducing heart disease. A vegan diet, which is cholesterol free, is best. Beans, of any type, are very effective at reducing blood cholesterol levels because of their content of soluble fiber. Soy beans have been extensively studied and are very helpful in reducing blood cholesterol and triglyceride levels. Other beans should have the same effect. *(American Journal of Clinical Nutrition, October 1983)* It would be a good idea to have dried beans, 3-4 times during the week. To prevent you from majoring in music, make sure you soak them overnight, rinse them several times, and cook them very slowly and for a long period of time. This will allow you to be more sociable and less musically incline.☺

Another excellent way to reduce LDL and total cholesterol is to use 1-2 tablespoons of ground flaxseed over your food at meals. I prefer it ground into a meal and sprinkled over my food each day. It has a slightly nutty taste, which I enjoy, especially in grits.☺

To improve your blood cholesterol profile, your diet should also contain at least 3-5 servings of vegetables and 3-5 servings of fruit each day. These foods contain fiber and are cholesterol free. Eat large quantities of whole grains, including: whole wheat, barley, rye, oats, brown rice, and corn. 6-11 servings should be eaten every day.

♦ **Temperance** - Tobacco and caffeine are both known risk factors for heart disease. Decaffeinated beverages may increase blood cholesterol levels. The belief that alcohol, particularly wine, is beneficial in reducing heart disease is incorrect. How can you help the heart and circulation, while you destroy brain and liver cells? Many promoting this approach are simply trying to justify their own use of this poisonous brew.

♦ **Water** - Because adequate hydration is important in preventing the blood from becoming too thick and sticky, 6-8 glasses of water should be consumed each day.

♦ **Air** - Deep breathing acts as a stress-reducer. I recommend three deep breaths, three times each day. If you exercise, you will breathe deeply.

♦ **Yielding Trust in God's Power** - *"Nay, in all these things we are more than conquerors through him that loved us." (Rom. 8:37)* The promise is that if you put your faith in Jesus, the changes necessary to prevent premature death from heart
disease will be made, through Jesus Christ.

Clinical Case #1 - A 48-year-old Black male with a 13-year history of diabetes, a risk factor for heart disease, comes in for a routine physical examination. Notice the impact of the BEST WAY program.

	Blood test 3/16/99	Repeat test 6/21/99
Cholesterol	237	204
Triglycerides	373	113
HDL Cholesterol	46	89
LDL Cholesterol	116	92
Chol./HDL Ratio	5.2	2.3
Glucose	186	98 (After med. reduced by 50%)

Clinical Case #2: A 51 year old Black male comes into the office for a routine physical examination. Blood chemistries are recorded below. The follow-up values were after the patient had been on the BEST WAY program for six weeks.

	Blood test 5/28/98	Blood test 7/13/98
Cholesterol	164	122
Triglycerides	567	296
HDL Cholesterol	25	23
LDL Cholesterol	26	40
Chl./HDL Cholesterol	6.6	5.3
Glucose	126	88

142

UPPER RESPIRATORY INFECTIONS
(The Common Cold)

Millions of Americans have this problem every year. Many, run to the doctor for medications which are of little or no benefit. Others use over-the-counter medications which may worsen the problem. The common cold is caused by over 200 different viruses; adenoviruses, RSV viruses, and rhinoviruses; the latter is the most common. Small children usually get 6-8 colds a year. They usually last for 1-2 weeks, and are destroyed by the body's immune system. Medications presently available will help to alleviate symptoms, but do not shorten the duration of the infection nor do they destroy the virus.

Symptoms include congestion in the head and chest, a runny nose, sore throat, low-grade fever (99-101°F), hoarseness, sneezing, coughing, muscle aches, and pain. Generalized fatigue may also be present. The runny nose is nature's way of fighting the infection. Mucus contains a natural virocidal, immunoglobulin A, which kills the viruses as the body expels them from the system. This is why antihistamines are to be avoided because they paralyze this defense mechanism by drying up the mucus and prolonging the time of recovery.

If your oral temperature rises above 103°F, or you have severe pain in the chest, head, abdomen or ears; or if there are enlarged lymph nodes in the neck, shortness of breath, or wheezing, you must seek medical attention promptly. You have more than a cold, a serious infection may be present.

What can be done to prevent colds? Taking a cool or tepid bath every day will help prevent colds, because it stimulates the immune response. Sleeping in a well-ventilated room prevents disease producing causing viruses from concentrating in your bedroom. Avoiding sweets and fatty foods is also very helpful. Have you noticed that many of these infections occur around the time we eat the most fats and sweets, Thanksgiving, Christmas, New Years, and Valentines Day?

In an effort to prevent the unnecessary use of medications and to help reduce your medical bills, find below several simple suggestions that will help in the treatment of colds. They will shorten the time it takes to recuperate from the infection.

1. Drink copious amounts of water, 8-10 glasses each day.

2. Run a humidifier or vaporizer continuously, but make sure it is cleaned as the manufacturer recommends.

3. Drink 2-3 cups of a mixture of red clover, peppermint and rose hips herbal tea. Honey or apple juice concentrate may be used as a sweetener.

4. Garlic and parsley tablets or capsules are also beneficial because of garlic's antiviral activity. Taking them before meals will allow you to be more sociable.☺ Echinacea may also be helpful.

5. Get plenty of rest! Lack of sleep is one of the most common causes for immune system compromise.

6. Mild exercise is beneficial. Vigorous exercise should be avoided.

7. Keep the room temperature between 65-75°F. Temperatures that are too high are not best in fighting viral infections.

8. Cool or hot baths are effective in stimulating the immune system. Using a heating compress is good for sore throats, as are charcoal tablets and warm salt water gargles.

9. Vick's Vapor Rub or its equivalent rubbed into the

chest at bedtime is helpful in suppressing the coughs associated with colds.

10. DO NOT take antibiotics unless the mucus becomes discolored, dark yellow, brown, or green. This may indicates that a bacterial infection is present. Antibiotics are effective in bacterial infections, but using them for viral infections only promotes the growth of resistant strains of bacteria.

Remember *Psalms 103:1-3, "Bless the LORD, O my soul: and all that is within me, bless his holy name. Bless the LORD, O my soul, and forget not all his benefits: Who forgiveth all thine iniquities; who health all thy diseases;"*

CONSTIPATION

Americans are "full of it."☺ We spend **$825,000,000** each year to treat constipation. *(Bonnie Liebman, Fiber, Nutrition Action Health Letter, Vol.21; No.7, Sept. 1994, p.6)* I have been in male restrooms and it sounded like I was in the labor and delivery room of a hospital because of the straining associated with this problem.☺

Constipation is physiologically associated with several serious conditions, including diverticulosis, diverticulitis, hemorrhoids and appendicitis. There are four causes of constipation, in most instances.
1. Inadequate water.
2. Inadequate fiber.
3. Lack of exercise.
4. Stress.

Any treatment approach which does not address each of these areas will not alleviate the problem. Common treatment options include, laxatives, colonics, or other unpleasant procedures, which I do not recommend.

As previously mentioned, flaxseed is an excellent source of fiber and is also inexpensive. You may also use psyllium or wheat bran. But if you don't get adequate water, these fiber sources will turn into "bricks," aggravating the problem. So here again, 6-8 glasses of water are recommended.

Walking for ten minutes after each meal is very effective not only in alleviating constipation, but also in aiding digestion.

If you follow these simple steps, you will be able to "move

freely," without discomfort, straining or other difficulties.

Clinical Case #1 - A 58-year-old Black female came into the office with a long history of digestive problems. They included, constipation, diarrhea, cramping, a bile or bitter taste in her mouth, abdominal bloating, nausea, and vomiting. The patient had undergone 9 abdominal surgeries in the past. Her abdomen resembled a "patch work quilt" with multiple healed surgical scars and moderate keloid formation. She was placed on the BEST WAY program. One month later on her follow-up visit, she reported that she was doing "much better." The bile taste and abdominal fullness had resolved. She no longer had abdominal cramping and was not constipated. The medications she was taking, which included a vegetarian enzyme complex, were stopped by the patient because she no longer needed them. She received relief, that only one month earlier, was not considered possible. One year after her initial visit finds the patient doing well! **WE THANK GOD FOR HIS BLESSINGS.**

CHAPTER 8

RATIONAL HERBAL & VITAMIN THERAPY

Herbal therapies have become increasingly popular in the past 10-15 years. More Americans are using more herbal and vitamin supplements than ever before. Between 35-40% of Americans admit to taking vitamin supplements regularly. *(The Wellness Encyclopedia, University of California, Berkeley, 1991; p.110)* One reason is because many believe the soil is so depleted of nutrients that they need to supplement their diets with vitamins. Vitamin deficiency diseases were a definite problem in past years. Pellagra, caused by an inadequate niacin intake; scurvy, induced by a vitamin C deficiency, and rickets due to a vitamin D deficiency are now rare. Even though they are more historical than actual problems today, they have spawned a multibillion dollar industry. Their toxicity when taken in large dosages is

148

not appreciated by many consumers, but they do exist. Let's look at the toxic effects of megadose vitamin supplementation.

Vitamin	Function	Sources	Toxicity
A	Night vision, bone and tooth formation, mucus secretions, epithelial integrity	Yellow and green vegetables. The deeper the color the more the vitamin A.	Stunting of growth, loss of appetite, dry skin, headaches, ringing in the ears, anemia, hair loss.
D	Bone & teeth formation, prevention of rickets.	Sunshine, animal fats	headaches, nausea, vomiting, diarrhea, reduced growth.
E	Antioxidant, retards aging	Widely distributed	Depression of bone calcification, increase in clotting time.
E	Blood coagulation (clotting)	Tomatoes, grains, cabbage, many others	Hemolytic anemia
B	Central nervous system function, skin integrity	Greens, beans, whole grains, fruit, vegetables.	Too much of one may cause imbalance of another.
C	Maintains collagen, cellular functions	Fruits, vegetables	GI irritant, vitamin balance, decrease copper metabolism
B-12	Blood formation, CNS function, GI function.	Greens, yeast, olives, soybeans, mouth bacteria, kelp, animal products	Cancer in animals in large dosages, increase seizures in seizure patients.

(Thrash, AM, Thrash, CL; Nutrition for Vegetarians, 1982, p.64-65)

What is the optimal dosage of these vitamins? What is the effect of the interaction of one vitamin on another? Will an overabundance of one interfere with another's activity? Does mineral supplementation cause a vitamin or mineral imbalance? The following lists shed light on the known interactions between different vitamins and minerals. This may help us to answer these questions.

VITAMIN INTERACTIONS

Vitamin A interacts with Vitamin E and Vitamin C.

Folacin interacts with Vitamins B, Vitamin B-12, Vitamin C.

Pantothenic Acid interacts with Vitamin B, niacin, riboflavin.

Vitamin B-6 interacts with Vitamin C, niacin, Vitamin B-12.

Biotin interacts with niacin, Vitamin B-12.

Vitamin E interacts with niacin, Vitamin C, Vitamin A.

Vitamin B-12 interacts with folacin, Vitamin B-6, biotin.

Riboflavin interacts with Pantothenic acid.

Niacin interacts with Pantothenic acid, Vitamin B-6, biotin, vitamin E.

Vitamin K interacts with Vitamin E.

Vitamin C interacts with Vitamin E, Vitamin B-6, folacin, Vitamin A.

Vitamins B interacts with pantothenic acid, folacin.

VITAMIN - MINERAL INTERACTIONS

Zinc interacts with Vitamin B-6, Folic acid, Vitamin A.

Vitamin D interacts with calcium, phosphorus.

Vitamin E interacts with selenium, zinc.

Vitamin C interacts with selenium, iron, copper.

Vitamin A interacts with zinc, calcium, iron.

Folic acid interacts with zinc.

Vitamin B-6 interacts with zinc.

Copper interacts with Vitamin C.

Iron interacts with Vitamin A, Vitamin C.

Phosphorus interacts with Vitamin D.

Calcium interacts with Vitamin A, Vitamin D.

Selenium interacts with Vitamin C, Vitamin E.

Nedley, Neil, M.D., Proof Positive: How to Reliably Combat Disease and Achieve Optimal Health through Nutrition and Lifestyle, 1998, p. 489

As you can see, these interactions have the potential for causing nutritional problems. This is more likely to occur when the supplements are taken individually and in high dosages. You may be doing yourself a great injustice by consuming large dosages of single or multiple vitamin supplements. If when reading the labels of these preparations, you see that the content is 10-20 times the recommended daily allowance (RDA); be careful. You should not use that supplement at all, or at least not on a regular basis.

One very interesting study showed that a high intake of beta-carotene, a precursor of vitamin A, caused a 16% increase of lung cancer in smokers, compared to smokers not taking the beta-carotene. But those using vitamin E supplements, had a 19% reduction in the incidence of lung cancer. Commenting on the study, Dr. Karen Woodson of the National Cancer Institute stated that taking vitamin E in a supplement form was not as effective in reducing lung cancer as was vitamin E obtained from food. *(Russ, C, Medical Tribune; Vol.40, Num.20, November 1999 No. II)*. It is not best to attempt to supplement specific nutrients randomly. A more appropriate course, in my opinion, would be to take a multivitamin and mineral tablet containing up to 100% of the RDA for each nutrient. This may be very helpful but, if it is not, at least it is not harmful.

If you have a medical condition, and are seeking the drug effect, and not the nutritional effect of the supplement, this is a "horse of a different color." A megadose vitamin or mineral supplement may be appropriate in that instance.

HERBS

Herbs are a big business. They have been purported to cure everything from cancer to diabetes to AIDS. But just what are they? Herbs are plants or parts of plants, which are extracted or dried. They are valued for their savory, aromatic, or medicinal qualities. *(The World Book Dictionary, 1989.)*

Not all herbs are safe. Note the following:

HERBS considered unsafe:

Arnica	Black cherry	Bloodroot
Buckthorn	Burdock root	Buttercups
Cohosh, blue	Comfrey	Elderberry
Foxglove	Goldenseal (too much)	Gordolobo
Jimsonweed	Kavakava	Lobelia
Mandrake	Marsh Marigold	Mate Melilot
Mormon tea	Nutmeg	Oleander
Pennyroyal	Periwinkle	Poke root
Rue	Sassafras	Snakeroot
Tansy Ragwort	Tonka bean	T's-san-chi
Water hemlock	Woodruff	Wormwood
Yohimbe bark	Skunk cabbage	

(Craig, WJ, The Use and Safety of Common Herbs and Herbal Teas, Golden Harvest Books, Second Edition, 1996, p.28-31).

Other herbs are of benefit in many medical conditions. Some are listed below.

WARNING: BEFORE USING HERBS TO TREAT MEDICAL PROBLEMS, PLEASE CONSULT WITH YOUR PHYSICIAN!

HERBS for Circulation

Ginkgo - helpful in the elderly for memory loss, absent-mindedness, anxiety, dizziness, headache, depression, confusion and other ailments. Helpful in early stages of ALZHEIMER'S DISEASE. Also helpful for circulatory conditions like atherosclerosis. DO NOT USE, IF YOU ARE TAKING A BLOOD THINNER.

Hawthorn berries - angina pectoris, blood clot prevention, and hypertension. This herb should not be used for any of the above conditions, without the approval of the patient's health care provider.

Psyllium - helps to lower cholesterol and is helpful in treating and preventing constipation. (1 teaspoon twice daily)

Flaxseed - lowers total and LDL, "lousy" cholesterol. Also has anti-inflammatory properties. Useful in treating and preventing constipation.

Garlic - regular use lowers total and LDL, "lousy" cholesterol. It lowers blood pressure and inhibits platelet aggregation, (helps to prevent premature clotting of the blood.)

Fenugreek - reduces LDL cholesterol and triglycerides. Reduces blood sugar in diabetics,

Anti-Cancer HERBS

The herbs below have the highest known anti-cancer properties:

Garlic	*Ginger*	*Licorice root*
Carrots	*Gotu kola*	

Those with modest cancer protective properties:

Onions	Flaxseed	Turmeric
Mints	Rosemary	Thyme
Oregano	Sage	Basil
Caraway	Dill	Lemon grass
Coriander	Fennel	Cherries

HERBS for the Nerves

Catnip	Gotu kola	Goldenseal
Hawthorn	*Hops*	Lemon balm
Valerian	*St. John's Wort*	Passion flower

HERBS for Headaches

Feverfew (Migraine)   *White willow Bark*
Lavender

HERBS for the Immune System

Echinacea	*Garlic*	Flaxseed
St. John's Wort	Licorice root	Hyssop

HERBS for Diabetics

Garlic	*Onions*	*Fenugreek seeds*
Gymnema	Spanish moss	*Dandelion root*
Juniper berries		

HERBS for the Prostate

Saw palmetto   *Stinging nettle*

HERBS for Digestion

Ginger (nausea)	Peppermint (IBS)
Chamomile	Turmeric(fat digestion)
Blueberries (Diarrhea)	Fresh blueberries
Fennel (indigestion)	

HERBS for the Kidneys

Diuretics: *Goldenrod*   Buchu   Juniper berries
            Parsley   Fennel

Infections: *Cranberries*   *Uva Ursi*   Goldenrod
            Buchu

HERBS for Coughs

Marshmallow root   Mullein flowers   Slippery Elm
Horehound   Anise   *Eucalyptus oil*
Fennel   *Thyme*   Licorice
Echinacea

HERBS for Pain

White willow bark   Chamomile   Hops
Mullein   Feverfew

(Craig, WJ, The Use and Safety of Common Herbs and Herbal Teas, Golden Harvest Books, Second Edition, 1996, p.42-64).

(ITALIC = VERY HELPFUL)

GUIDELINES FOR THE SAFE USE OF HERB TEAS

1. Refrain from considering herbal beverages as natural panaceas.
2. Be alert to the toxicity of certain herbs.
3. Beware of unlabeled "loose" or bulk teas.
4. Read labels carefully so that only prepackaged teas with safe ingredients are used.
5. Use only those teas with safe constituents. For minor ailments use these teas in a therapeutic, not in a preventive or prophylactic fashion.
6. Drink only 1-2 cups of tea per day on a regular basis since the long term effect of drinking most herb teas in large quantities is not known.
7. People who show allergic response to ragweed, asters, or chrysanthemums should avoid all teas containing marigold, yarrow, and chamomile flowers.
8. Pregnant women should use caution in using any herbal teas, since few have been thoroughly tested for safety. Young children should also be cautious in using herbal teas.
9. **Herbal teas should not be used as a substitute for competent medical care.**
10. Do not use herbal preparations containing more than four herbs in them regularly.

(Craig, WJ, The Use and Safety of Common Herbs and Herbal Teas, Golden Harvest Books, Second Edition, 1996, p.27).

CHAPTER 9

TOTAL HEALTH, YOURS FOR THE ASKING!

Ask, and it shall be given you; seek, and ye shall find; knock, and it shall be opened unto you: For every one that asketh receiveth; and he that seeketh findeth; and to him that knocketh it shall be opened. Or what man is there of you, whom if his son ask bread, will he give him a stone? Or if he ask a fish, will give him a serpent? If ye then, being evil, know how to give good gifts unto your children, how much more shall you Father which is in heaven give good things to them that ask him? (Matthew 7:7-12)

God loves all of His children and that includes you! He paid an infinite price on Calvary's cross so that you and I might have the abundant life that comes only through Him. God

157

wants us to be healthy. This is shown by the fact that Jesus spent more time healing, during His earthly ministry, than He did preaching. He says in the third epistle of John, *"Beloved, I wish above all things, that thou mayest prosper and be in health, even as thy soul prospereth." (3 John 2)*

But the fact remains, many in our world are sick, maybe even you! Factors such as genetics and environmental conditions, contribute to the illnesses that we suffer. But the primary factor that is responsible for the "lion's share" of the chronic diseases in our society today, is LIFESTYLE! God is the source of all health, mental, physical, and spiritual. But He is unable to do for us what He desires, without our cooperation. He never forces His will upon us. It must be a Divine-human partnership.

God's Word is full of promises, such as, *"And said, If thou wilt diligently hearken to the voice of the Lord thy God, and wilt do that which is right in his sight, and wilt give ear to commandments, and keep all his statutes, I will put none of these diseases upon thee, which I have brought upon the Egyptians: for I am the Lord that healeth thee." (Exodus 15:26)* What were the diseases that plagued the Egyptians? Paleopathologists, those who study diseases of ancient civilizations tell us that the Egyptians were plagued by hypertension, heart disease, diabetes, obesity, arthritis, tooth decay, cancer, and others. These same diseases are very prevalent today! Are you diligently hearkening to God's voice? Or do you hearken only when it's convenient?

The Word of God also says, *" . . . Behold, to obey is better than sacrifice, and to hearken than the fat of rams." (1 Samuel 15:22)* Obedience is the only way to demonstrate that

God is # 1 in your life. It is the only way to show that you truly love your Saviour who has done everything possible, to give you health, peace, joy, and contentment.

In an effort to galvanize this principle in your mind and heart, I quote the words of Jesus Himself, when He said, *"If ye love me, keep my commandments" (John 14:15)*. Obedience is the fruit that grows on the tree of love! Gary Michael Davis, M.D., a friend of mine once said, while we were in medical school, "The only appropriate response to love, is love!"

Because of God's love for us, in His Word, He has given you and I principles of health. Do you remember the incident in the Bible when the ten lepers came to Jesus desiring to be healed of their leprosy? Jesus told them to go and show themselves to the priest, and the Bible records, " . . . *And it came to pass, that, as they went, they were cleansed." (Luke 17:14)* As they were obedient to the command of the Saviour, they were healed. I believe that this is one of the ways Jesus works today.

Several clinical cases have been previously shared, that show that with God, all things are possible. Many of the results I see in my practice, I cannot explain from a purely medical prospective. I **KNOW** the results are due to the intervention of God and the cooperation of His beloved children. This is why no patient leaves my office before we have prayed, unless they refuse. God always hears and answers prayer according to His will. Your part is to choose to follow God; choose to live-out in your life, the light that shines on your path, in the area of health, and in all the other areas of your life. If you don't choose God's way, the "BEST WAY," then you are by default, choosing the way of the enemy. And

Satan's way leads to disease, misery, and premature death. If we will do the things we know we should, then, with God's blessings, optimal health will surely be ours.

But now to put things in their proper prospective. If you choose Jesus, you are choosing health! He is the source of health, He is the power to carry out the instructions He has given. He is the, I AM, everything you need. So stop majoring in minors. *"But seek you first the kingdom of God, and his righteousness; and all these things shall be added unto you."* *(Matthew 6:33).* So before you do anything else, make sure you have spent time with the Saviour. Then, the struggle to eat correctly, exercise regularly, and get proper sleep, will not be so overwhelming. These things shall be added unto you, when you put Jesus first!

Over the course of this short book I have attempted, through the aid of the Holy Spirit, to share some of God's principles of health. My appeal and prayer for you is that you give your heart unreservedly, to our kind and compassionate Creator and Saviour, Jesus Christ. For this truly is *"YOUR BEST WAY TO HEALTH!"*

Dr. Moore's Top 20 Recipes
Breakfast

Scrambled Tofu

1-1 lb. Tofu-mashed	1 t. yeast flakes
1 T. chicken style seasoning	1/4 t. garlic powder
½ t. onion powder	1/4 t. turmeric
½ t. salt	1/4 diced onion or 1 T. dried onion

Put all of the ingredients in a skillet, stirring well. Cook for 20 minutes, and until a vibrant yellow color. May add green and red peppers.

Plain Granola

In a large bowl, mix well:

7 c. oats	3/4 c wheat germ
½ c. oat bran	

In a blender, mix well:

½ c. oil	1 T. vanilla
1/3 c. sweetener	1 t. salt
½ c. warm water	1 t. coriander

Add to dry mixture, mix well with your hands. Bake at 150° degrees for about 3 hours.

Potato Cakes

5 washed unpeeled potatoes-cubed and cooked until tender.

Add: ½ c. soy milk	2 T. oil
1 ½ t. onion powder	1 ½ T. parsley flakes
1 ½ t. chicken seasoning	1 t. salt

Mash and mix all ingredients well. Spoon onto oiled pan. Bake at 375° for 20 minutes on each side.

Taken from Country Life Cookbook

Waffles

In a blender:

2 c. hot water ½ c. cashews

1 c oats ½ t. salt

1/3 c. sweetener

Dissolve in a small bowl:

½ t. yeast 1/4 c. water

In a large bowl add blended mixture, then yeast mixture. Then add: 1 ½ c. unbleached white flour ½ c. whole wheat flour

1/4 c. oil 1 ½ T. vanilla

Add maple or other flavoring as desired.

Place in waffle iron and cook for 8-10 minutes.

Apple Syrup

In a blender:

1 - 6 oz. can frozen apple 1 - 6 oz. can water

4 t. cornstarch ½ t. lemon juice

1/4 t. coriander

Pour into pan and cook over low heat to the desired thickness

Taken from Country Life Cookbook

Fruit Crisp

Drain: 2 - 29 oz. can of sliced peaches or 3 - 4 sliced apples in 1 c pineapple juice. Sprinkle with raisins. Put in baking dish.

Topping : 1/4 c. oil 1/4 c. honey

1/4 c. water ½ t. salt

1 t. coriander 1 t. vanilla

2 3/4 c. rolled oat 1/4 c. flour

Bake at 350° for 25 minutes.

Taken from Country Life Cookbook

Main Entree's

Spaghetti Primavera

Stir fry approx. 2 C. of California blend with onions and 1 can drained mushrooms.
In a pot:

2 cans of tomato sauce	½ t. onion powder
1/4 t. Italian seasoning	½ t. parsley
1/4 t. salt	

Heat thoroughly. Serve vegetables atop sauce atop noodles.

Chickpea a la King

Blend:

1 c. cooked garbanzos	1/4 c. flour
3 T. chicken-like seasoning	3 c. water
½ t. salt	½ c cashews
4 t. sesame seeds	

Saute:

1 med. onion, chopped with 1- 4 oz. can mushroom.

Heat blended mixture and add 1 c. green peas and sauteed mixture.

Cook pasta (flat noodles). Fold all ingredients together. Bake at 350° for 20 minutes

Rice Patties

Saute:

½ c. chopped onions	½ c. chopped celery
1/4 c. yeast flakes	2 T. oil
1/8 t. garlic salt	½ t. salt
1 T. chicken-like seasoning	2 T. Brag's Aminos
½ c. chopped almonds	2 c. cooked brown rice

Mix well then add 2 c. shredded potatoes. Spoon patties onto oiled pan. Bake at 350° for about 20 minutes each side or 40 minutes on one side. Let cool before removing.

Oatburgers

2 1/4 c. water	½ chopped onion
½ c. Brag's Aminos	½ T. basil
½ T. oregano	½ T. onion powder
1/8 t. garlic powder	1/8 c. yeast flakes
½ T. chicken-like seasoning	½ c. gluten

Bring to a boil then add 2 1/4 c. oats. Turn off heat and let sit for 15 minutes after stirring well. Form into patties on oiled pan. Bake at 350° for about 20 minutes each side.

Pam's Pizza
(2 large round)

Dough:

2 1/4 c. warm water   3/4 c. mashed potatoes
1 ½ T. yeast   1 ½ T. sweetener

Mix and let rise for 10 minutes.

Then add:

8 c. flour (mixture unbleached and whole wheat)
2 t. salt   1/3 c. oil

Knead, then roll into pizza crust shape.

Add a layer of your favorite spaghetti sauce.
Then add a layer of cashew pimento cheese sauce. (See below)

Top with chopped vegetables such as:

Mushrooms, Olives, Green, red, yellow peppers, Onion, Olives, etc. and a soy-based meat substitutes if desired.

Bake in oven for approximately 20-25 minutes at 350°F.

NOTE: For thicker crust, let dough rise before adding toppings.

Cashew Pimento Cheeze

Blend until smooth:

1 (4 oz. jar pimentos) 3 T. yeast flakes   3/4 c. cashews
1 t. onion powder   2 T. sesame seeds   1 t. salt
1/8 t. garlic powder   1/4 c. lemon juice   1 c. water

Beefy Lasagna

3/4 lb. Veggie meat
1 c. chopped onion
2 cloves minced garlic
1- 8 oz. can tomato sauce
1- 7 oz. can tomato paste
½ c. Vegan Parmesan cheese

1 T. Italian seasoning
½ t. salt
1- 8 oz. pkg. of tofu
1 egg substitute
1 T. parsley

Brown veggie meat with onions and garlic.

Stir in tomato sauce, tomato paste, Italian seasoning and salt. Cook for 15 minutes.

Mash tofu and stir in egg substitute, ½ of the Parmesan cheese and parsley flakes.

Arrange noodles. Top with ½ tofu filling. Then half of meat sauce and cheese substitute. Repeat with second layer.

Sprinkle top with remaining Parmesan cheese. Bake at 375° for 30 minutes. Let stand 10 minutes before serving.

Desserts

Yomi's Carob Covered Nutty Granola

2 c. bag carob chip	½ c. peanut butter
½ c. raisins	1 t. vanilla
½ c. coconut	½ c. honey
2 c. granola	

Melt carob and peanut butter. Add remaining ingredients (may need to add a little milk) Chill and cut in squares.

Carob Fudge Brownies

Mix together: ½ c honey	1/3 c oil
2 T. dry sweetener	½ t. salt
1 t. vanilla	1 t. lemon juice
½ c. soy milk	½ c. carob powder
1/4 c. pecans	1 c. flour

Pour batter in baking dish. Bake at 350° for 25-30 minutes.

Taken from Favorite Wildwood Recipes

Crumb Topped Peach Pie with Pecan Pastry

Filling: 2 c. sliced peaches	1/4 c. Sucanat
3 T. flour	1/4 t. coriander

Mix dry ingredients first, the add to peaches.

Pastry: 1 1/4 c. flour	1/4 t. salt
1/3 c. oil with 3 T. water	1/4 c. chopped pecans

Mix oil and water together first. Add remaining ingredients. Mix well and roll between waxed paper.

Topping: 1/4 c. flour	2 T. Sucanat or brown sugar.
1 T. soy margarine	

Mix in flour and Sucanat. Cut in soy margarine.
Sprinkle over peaches. Bake 375° for 25 minutes.

Tofu Cheese Cake

In a blender whiz:

1 lb. mashed tofu	3 T. vanilla
3/4 c. honey	½ t. salt
½ c. oil	1 t. lemon flavoring
3 T. lemon juice	1 t. maple flavoring
Crust: 3 c. ground granola	3 T. oil
2 t. coriander	2 T. honey
1 T. water	

Press crust into baking dish and pour blended mixture over top. Bake at 350° for 20 minutes.

Fruit Topping: In a sauce pan add ½ c. water and 3 T. cornstarch. Bring to a boil, cook 1 minute. Add berries and sweetener if needed. Cook 1 minute more, coating fruit well. Spread over cooled baked tofu and crust. Chill.

Taken from Country Life Cookbook

Apple Pie with Oat Crust

Filling: 6 c. sliced, un-peeled apples and 3/4 c. frozen apple juice concentrated (unsweetened) simmered over heat for about 5 minutes.

Mix together:

2 T. water	1/8 t. salt
2 T. cornstarch	½ t. coriander

Add to apples. Cook 1 minute.

Crust: Top and bottom	
1 c. oat flour	½ c. oil
1 c. unbleached flour	½ c. cold water
1 t. salt	

Bake at 350° for about 40 minutes.

Miscellaneous

Tofu Greek Salad

1 lb. cubed tofu cooked (boiled) in 2 c. water seasoned with 3 T. chicken like seasoning. Drain and let cool.

Then mix together:

½ c. oil	2 cubed tomatoes
1/4 c. lemon juice	½ c. chopped onions
½ T. salt	1 t. basil
½ t. oregano	Black olives

Add to cubed tofu.

Apple Brown Betty

In a medium bowl, stir together.

3-4 cubed apples with skin	2 T. sweetener
1 t. lemon juice	1/4 c. raisins
pinch of salt	

Then put the mixture in a baking dish.
In same bowl mix well the following.

3-4 slices bread-cubed	½ c. wheat germ
1 T. oil	

Add to cover apple mixture.
Bake at 350° for 25 minutes.

Taken from Favorite Wildwood Recipes

Health Age Appraisal
Longevity and Lifestyle

Drs. Breslow and Belloc's of UCLA identified seven health factors which impacted health and longevity.

1. Getting 7 - 8 hours of sleep each day.
2. Not eating between meals.
3. Eating breakfast regularly.
4. Maintaining proper weight.
5. Getting regular exercise.
6. Moderate or NO use of alcohol.
7. Not smoking.

The chart below shows an inverse relationship between health habits and the risk of premature death. (The greater the number of positive health habits practiced, the lower the death rate.)

Relationship of Longevity to Health Habits Age-adjusted death rate		
No. of health habits practiced	Percent dead in 9 years MEN	Percent dead in 9 years WOMEN
7	5.5	5.3
6	11.0	7.7
5	13.4	8.2
4	14.1	10.8
0 - 3	20.0	12.3

(For a longer life, the BEST WAY is the best way!)

The Health Age Appraisal

How old are you, really? You can determine your health age by finding how many of the seven health factors you practice. Then find your age and add or subtract the number below to or from your chronological age. (Example: I am 45 years old and I practice all seven health habits, therefore I would subtract 12.9 years from my age. This would give me the health age of 32.1 years. I'M YOUNGER THAN MANY THINK! HOW OLD ARE YOU, REALLY?☺

HEALTH AGE RELATED TO LIFESTYLE HABITS (For men and women)						
Age	Habits 0-2	Habits 3	Habits 4	Habits 5	Habits 6	Habits 7
20	+14.3	+7.4	+0.5	-1.1	-4.2	-9.4
30	+16.9	+9.1	+3.0	-0.6	-4.7	-11.1
40	+19.4	+10.7	+5.4	-0.1	-5.2	-12.9
50	+22.0	+12.4	+7.9	+0.3	-5.7	-14.7
60	+24.5	+14.0	+10.4	+0.8	-6.2	-16.4
70	+27.1	+15.7	+12.8	+1.3	-6.8	-18.2

How did you fair? If you did not do that well, do not fret. By submitting to God and choosing to make changes in your health habits, you can become "younger."

For More Information:

If you are interested in rational natural medical treatment, copies of this book, or would like Dr. Moore to speak for your church, civic organization or health group, please contact him at:

> *BEST WAY to Health, Inc.*
> *PO Box 463*
> *Conyers, GA 30012*
> *770-761-6349 or email us at: bestwaytohealth@yahoo.com*

Reading Resources

The Holy Bible

Country Life Cookbook
> Edited by Diana Fleming, Family Health Publications, 1990

Get Well at Home
> Richard A. Hansen, MD, Shiloh Medical Publications, 1980

Ministry of Healing
> Ellen G. White, Pacific Press Publishing, 1905

Plus 15 Plan for Health Enhancement 15 Days to Lower Blood Pressure and Cholesterol, Samuel L. DeShay, MD, and Bernice A. DeShay, RN, Upward Way Inc. 1990

Proof Positive, How to Reliably Combat Disease and Achieve Optimal Health through Nutrition and Lifestyle, Neil Nedley, MD, Nedley Publishers, 1998, Ardmore, OK

Somethin' To Shout About!
> Donna Green-Goodman, MPH, Orion Enterprises, 1999 *The*

TEMPERANCE PLEDGE

I do on this day choose to live a temperate life, by the grace of our Lord and Savior Jesus Christ. I do pledge that whether I eat or drink or whatsoever I do, I will do all to the glory of God!

For Jesus Sake, Amen!

_____   _____
Signed   Date

NOTES

NOTES

NOTES